2012

GUIDE FOR AVIATION MEDICAL EXAMINERS

Welcome to the Guide for Aviation Medical Examiners. The format of this version of the Guide provides instant access to information regarding regulations, medical history, examination procedures, disposition, and protocols, necessary for completion of the FAA Form 8500-8, Application for Airman Medical Certificate or Airman Medical and Student Pilot Certificate.

To navigate through the Guide PDF by Item number or subject matter, simply click on the "BOOKMARK" tab in the left column to search specific certification decision-making criteria. To expand any "BOOKMARK" files, click on the corresponding + button located in the front of the text. To collapse any of the expanded files, click on the + button again.

The most current version of this guide may be found and downloaded at the following FAA site:

http://www.faa.gov/about/office_org/headquarters_offices/avs/offices/aam/ame/guide/

LAST UPDATE: December 14, 2012

TABLE OF CONTENTS

Forms: http://www.faa.gov/library/forms

Federal Aviation Administration
  Regional and Center Medical Office Addresses:

http://www.faa.gov/licenses_certificates/medical_certification/rfs

Federal Aviation Administration
  FAA Flight Standards District Offices (FSDO's):

http://www.faa.gov/about/office_org/field_offices/fsdo

Title 14 Code of Federal Regulations
  Part 67 — Medical Standards and Certification:

http://ecfr.gpoaccess.gov/

Convention on International Civil Aviation
  International Standards on Personnel Licensing:

The international Standards on Personnel Licensing are contained in Annex 1 – *Personnel Licensing* to the Convention on International Civil Aviation. The FAA maintains an updated, hard copy of all the ICAO Annexes and also an on-line subscription. The FAA makes copies of Annex 1 available at seminars and can provide Examiner's access upon request.

http://www.dfld.de/Downloads/Annex_01.pdf

GENERAL INFORMATION

This section provides input to assist an Aviation Medical Examiner (AME), otherwise known as an Examiner, in performing his or her duties in an efficient and effective manner. It also describes Examiner responsibilities as the Federal Aviation Administration's (FAA) representative in medical certification matters and as the link between airmen and the FAA.

1. Legal Responsibilities of Designated Aviation Medical Examiners

Title 49, United States Code (U.S.C.) (Transportation), sections 109(9), 40113(a), 44701-44703, and 44709 (1994) formerly codified in the Federal Aviation Act of 1958, as amended, authorizes the FAA Administrator to delegate to qualified private persons; i.e. designated Examiners, matters related to the examination, testing, and inspection necessary to issue a certificate under the U.S.C. and to issue the certificate. Designated Examiners are delegated the Administrator's authority to examine applicants for airman medical certificates and to issue or deny issuance of certificates.

Approximately 450,000 applications for airman medical certification are received and processed each year. The vast majority of medical examinations conducted in connection with these applications are performed by physicians in private practice who have been designated to represent the FAA for this purpose. An Examiner is a designated representative of the FAA Administrator with important duties and responsibilities. It is essential that Examiners recognize the responsibility associated with their appointment.

At times, an applicant may not have an established treating physician and the Examiner may elect to fulfill this role. You must consider your responsibilities in your capacity as an Examiner as well as the potential conflicts that may arise when performing in this dual capacity.

The consequences of a negligent or wrongful certification, which would permit an unqualified person to take the controls of an aircraft, can be serious for the public, for the Government, and for the Examiner. If the examination is cursory and the Examiner fails to find a disqualifying defect that should have been discovered in the course of a thorough and careful examination, a safety hazard may be created and the Examiner may bear the responsibility for the results of such action.

Of equal concern is the situation in which an Examiner deliberately fails to report a disqualifying condition either observed in the course of the examination or otherwise known to exist. In this situation, both the applicant and the Examiner in completing the application and medical report form may be found to have committed a violation of Federal criminal law which provides that:

> "Whoever in any matter within the jurisdiction of any department or agency of the United States knowingly and willfully falsifies, conceals, or covers up by any trick, scheme, or device a material fact, or who makes any false, fictitious or fraudulent statements or representations, or entry, may be fined up to $250,000 or imprisoned not more than 5 years, or both" (Title 18 U.S. Code. Secs. 1001; 3571).

Cases of falsification may be subject to criminal prosecution by the Department of Justice. This is true whether the false statement is made by the applicant, the Examiner, or both. In view of the pressures sometimes placed on Examiners by their regular patients to ignore a disqualifying physical defect that the physician knows to exist, it is important that all Examiners be aware of possible consequences of such conduct.

In addition, when an airman has been issued a medical certificate that should not have been issued, it is frequently necessary for the FAA to begin a legal revocation or suspension action to recover the certificate. This procedure is time consuming and costly. Furthermore, until the legal process is completed, the airman may continue to exercise the privileges of the certificate, thereby compromising aviation safety.

2. Authority of Aviation Medical Examiners

The Examiner is delegated authority to:

- Examine applicants for, and holders of, airman medical certificates to determine whether or not they meet the medical standards for the issuance of an airman medical certificate.

- Issue or deny airman medical certificates to applicants or holders of such certificates based upon whether or not they meet the applicable medical standards. The medical standards are found in Title 14 of the Code of Federal Regulations, part 67.

A medical certificate issued by an Examiner is considered to be affirmed as issued unless, within 60 days after date of issuance (date of examination), it is reversed by the Federal Air Surgeon, a RFS, or the Manager, AMCD. However, if the FAA requests additional information from the applicant within 60 days after the issuance, the above-named officials have 60 days after receipt of the additional information to reverse the issuance.

3. Equipment Requirements

For the conduct of the medical examination, Examiners shall have adequate facilities for performing the required examinations and possess the following equipment prior to conducting any FAA examinations. History or current findings may indicate a need for special evaluations. Examiners shall certify at the time of designation, re-designation, or upon request that they possess (and maintain as necessary) the equipment specified.

1. Standard Snellen Test. Types for visual acuity (both near and distant) and appropriate eye lane. FAA Form 8500-1, Near Vision Acuity Test Card may be used for near and intermediate vision testing. Metal, opaque plastic, or cardboard occluder.

2. Eye Muscle Test-Light. May be a spot of light 0.5cm in diameter, a regular muscle-test light, or an ophthalmoscope.

3. Maddox Rod. May be hand-type.

4. Horizontal Prism Bar. Risley or hand prism are acceptable alternatives.

5. Other vision test equipment that is acceptable as a replacement for 1 through 4 above include any commercially available visual acuities and heterophoria testing devices.

6. Color Vision Test Apparatus. Pseudoisochromatic plates, (American Optical Company (AOC), l965 edition; AOC-HRR, 2nd edition); Dvorine, 2nd edition; Ishihara, Concise 14 -, 24 -, or 38-plate editions; or Richmond (l983 edition, 15-plates). Acceptable substitutes are: Farnsworth Lantern; OPTEC 900 Color Vision Test; Keystone Orthoscope; Keystone Telebinocular; LKC Technologies, Inc., Apt-5 Color Vision Tester; OPTEC 2000 Vision Tester (Models 2000 PM, 2000 PAME, 2000 PI); OPTEC 2500; Titmus Vision Tester; Titmus II Vision Tester (Model Nos. TII and TIIS); Titmus 2 Vision Tester (Models T2A and T2S); Titmus i400.

7. A Wall Target consisting of a 50-inch square surface with a matte finish (may be black felt or dull finish paper) and a 2-mm white test object (may be a pin) in a suitable handle of the same color as the background. Note: this is not necessary if an AME chooses the acceptable option of performing field of vision testing by direct confrontation.

8. Standard physician diagnostic instruments and aids including those necessary to perform urine testing for albumin and glucose and those to measure height and weight.

9. Electrocardiographic equipment. Senior Examiners must have access to digital electrocardiographic equipment with electronic transmission capability.

10. Audiometric equipment. All Examiners must have access to audiometric equipment or a capability of referring applicants to other medical facilities for audiometric testing.

4. Medical Certification Decision Making

The format of the Guide establishes aerospace medical dispositions, protocols, and AME Assisted Special Issuances (AASI) identified in Items 21–58 of the FAA Form 8500. This guidance references specific medical tests or procedure(s) the results of which are needed by the FAA to determine the eligibility of the applicant to be medically certificated. The request for this medical information must not be misconstrued as the FAA ordering or mandating that the applicant undergo testing, where clinically inappropriate or contraindicated. The risk of the study based upon the disease state and test conditions must be balanced by the applicant's desire for certification and determined by the applicant and their healthcare provider(s).

After reviewing the medical history and completing the examination, Examiners must:

- Issue a medical certificate,

- Deny the application, or

- Defer the action to the Manager, AMCD, AAM-300, or the appropriate RFS

Examiners **may issue** a medical certificate *only* if the applicant meets all medical standards, including those pertaining to medical history unless otherwise authorized by the FAA.

Examiners **may not issue** a medical certificate if the applicant fails to meet specified minimum standards or demonstrates any of the findings or diagnoses described in this Guide as "disqualifying" unless the condition is unchanged or improved and the applicant presents written documentation that the FAA has evaluated the condition, found the applicant eligible for certification, and authorized Examiners to issue certificates. The following medical conditions are specifically disqualifying under 14 CFR part 67. However, the FAA may exercise discretionary authority under the provisions of Authorization of Special Issuance, to issue an airman medical certificate. See **Special Issuances** section for additional guidance where applicable.

- Angina pectoris;

- Bipolar disorder;

- Cardiac valve replacement;

- Coronary heart disease that has required treatment or, if untreated, that has been symptomatic or clinically significant;

- Diabetes mellitus requiring insulin or other hypoglycemic medication;

- Disturbance of consciousness without satisfactory medical explanation of the cause;

- Epilepsy;

- Heart replacement;

- Myocardial infarction;

- Permanent cardiac pacemaker;

- Personality disorder that is severe enough to have repeatedly manifested itself by overt acts;

- Psychosis;

- Substance abuse and dependence;

- Transient loss of control of nervous system function(s) without satisfactory medical explanation of cause.

An airman who is medically disqualified for any reason may be considered by the FAA for an Authorization for Special Issuance of a Medical Certificate (Authorization). For medical defects, which are static or nonprogressive in nature, a Statement of Demonstrated Ability (SODA) may be granted in lieu of an Authorization.

The Examiner **always may defer** the application to the FAA for action. In the interests of the applicant and of a responsive certification system, however, deferral is appropriate only if the standards are not met; if there is an unresolved question about the history, the findings, the standards, or agency policy; if the examination is incomplete; if further evaluation is necessary; or if directed by the FAA.

The Examiner may deny certification *only* when the applicant clearly does not meet the standards.

5. Authorization for Special Issuance and AME Assisted Special Issuance (AASI)

A. Authorization for Special Issuance of a Medical Certificate (Authorization).

At the discretion of the Federal Air Surgeon, an Authorization for Special Issuance of a Medical Certificate (Authorization), valid for a specified period, may be granted to a person who does not meet the established medical standards if the person shows to the satisfaction of the Federal Air Surgeon that the duties authorized by the class of medical certificate applied for can be performed without endangering public safety during the period in which the Authorization would be in force. The Federal Air Surgeon may authorize a special medical flight test, practical test, or medical evaluation for this purpose. A medical certificate of the appropriate class may be issued to a person who fails to meet one or more of the established medical standards if that person possesses a valid agency issued Authorization and is otherwise eligible. An airman medical certificate issued in accordance with the special issuance section of part 67 (14 CFR § 67.401), shall expire no later than the end of the validity period or upon the withdrawal of the Authorization upon which it is based. An airman must again show to the satisfaction of the Federal Air Surgeon that the duties authorized by the class of medical certificate applied for can be performed without endangering public safety in order to obtain a new medical certificate and/or a Re-Authorization.

In granting an Authorization, the Federal Air Surgeon may consider the person's operational experience and any medical facts that may affect the ability of the person to perform airman duties including:

- The factors leading to and surrounding the episode

- The combined effect on the person of failing to meet one or more than one requirement of part 67; and

- The prognosis derived from professional consideration of all available information regarding the person

In granting an Authorization, the Federal Air Surgeon specifies the class of medical certificate authorized to be issued and may do any or all of the following:

- Limit the duration of an Authorization;

- Condition the granting of a new Authorization on the results of subsequent medical tests, examinations, or evaluations;

- State on the Authorization, and any medical certificate based upon it, any operational limitation needed for safety; or

- Condition the continued effect of an Authorization, and any second- or third-class medical certificate based upon it, on compliance with a statement of functional limitations issued to the person in coordination with the Director of Flight Standards or the Director's designee

- In determining whether an Authorization should be granted to an applicant for a third-class medical certificate, the Federal Air Surgeon considers the freedom of an airman, exercising the privileges of a private pilot certificate, to accept reasonable risks to his or her person and property that are not acceptable in the exercise of commercial or airline transport pilot privileges, and, at the same time, considers the need to protect the safety of persons and property in other aircraft and on the ground

An Authorization granted to a person who does not meet the applicable medical standards of part 67 may be withdrawn, at the discretion of the Federal Air Surgeon, at any time if:

- There is adverse change in the holder's medical condition;

- The holder fails to comply with a statement of functional limitations or operational limitations issued as a condition of certification under the special issuance section of part 67 (14 CFR 67.401);

- Public safety would be endangered by the holder's exercise of airman privileges;

- The holder fails to provide medical information reasonably needed by the Federal Air Surgeon for certification under the special issuance section of part 67 (14 CFR 67.401); or

- The holder makes or causes to be made a statement or entry that is the basis for withdrawal of an Authorization under the falsification section of part 67 (14 CFR 67.403)

A person who has been granted an Authorization under the special issuance section of part 67 (14 CFR 67.401), based on a special medical flight or practical test, need not take the test again during later medical examinations unless the Federal Air Surgeon determines or has reason to believe that the physical deficiency has or may have degraded to a degree to require another special medical flight test or practical test.

The authority of the Federal Air Surgeon under the special issuance section of part 67 (14 CFR 67.401) is also exercised by the Manager, AMCD, and each RFS.

If an Authorization is withdrawn at any time, the following procedures apply:

- The holder of the Authorization will be served a letter of withdrawal, stating the reason for the action;

- By not later than 60 days after the service of the letter of withdrawal, the holder of the Authorization may request, in writing, that the Federal Air Surgeon provide for review of the decision to withdraw. The request for review may be accompanied by supporting medical evidence;

- Within 60 days of receipt of a request for review, a written final decision either affirming or reversing the decision to withdraw will be issued; and

- A medical certificate rendered invalid pursuant to a withdrawal, in accordance with the special issuance section of part 67 (14 CFR 67.401) shall be surrendered to the Administrator upon request

B. AME Assisted Special Issuance (AASI).

AME Assisted Special Issuance (AASI) is a process that provides Examiners the ability to re-issue an airman medical certificate under the provisions of an Authorization to an applicant who has a medical condition that is disqualifying under 14 CFR part 67. An FAA physician provides the initial certification decision and grants the Authorization in accordance with 14 CFR § 67.401. The Authorization letter is accompanied by attachments that specify the information that treating physician(s) must provide for the re-issuance determination. Examiners may re-issue an airman medical certificate under the provisions of an Authorization, if the applicant provides the requisite medical information required for determination. Examiners may not issue initial Authorizations. An Examiner's decision or determination is subject to review by the FAA.

6. Privacy of Medical Information

A. Within the FAA, access to an individual's medical information is strictly on a "need-to-know" basis. The safeguards of the Privacy Act apply to the application for airman medical certification and to other medical files in the FAA's possession. The FAA does not release medical information without an order from a court of competent jurisdiction, written permission from the individual to whom it applies, or, with the individual's knowledge, during litigation of matters related to certification. The FAA does, however, on request, disclose the fact that an individual holds an airman medical certificate and its class, and it may provide medical information regarding a pilot involved in an accident to the National Transportation Safety Board (NTSB) (or to a physician of the appropriate medical discipline who is retained by the NTSB for use in aircraft accident investigation.)

The Examiner, as a representative of the FAA, should treat the applicant's medical certification information in accordance with the requirements of the Privacy Act. Therefore, information should not be released without the written consent of the applicant or an order from a court of competent jurisdiction. In order to ensure that release of information is proper, whenever a court order or subpoena is received by the Examiner, the appropriate RFS, or the AMCD, should be contacted. Similarly, unless the applicant's written consent for release is of a routine nature; e.g., accompanying a standard insurance company request, advice should be sought from the FAA before releasing any information. In all cases, copies of all released information should be retained.

B. Health Insurance Portability and Accountability Act of 1996 (HIPAA) and Examiner's activities for the FAA. This Act provides specific patient protections and depending upon an Examiner's activation and practice patterns, you may have to comply with additional requirements.

C. Examiners shall certify at the time of designation, re-designation, or upon request that they shall protect the privacy of medical information.

7. Release of Information

Except in compliance with an order of a court of competent jurisdiction, or upon an applicant's written request, Examiners will not divulge or release copies of any reports prepared in connection with the examination to anyone other than the applicant or the FAA. A copy of the examination may be released to the applicant upon request. Upon receipt of a court subpoena or order, the Examiner shall notify the appropriate RFS. Other requests for information will be referred to:

MANAGER
AEROSPACE MEDICAL CERTIFICATION DIVISION, AAM-331
CIVIL AEROMEDICAL INSTITUTE
FEDERAL AVIATION ADMINISTRATION
POST OFFICE BOX 26200
OKLAHOMA CITY, OK 73125-0080

8. No "Alternate" Examiners Designated

The Examiner is to conduct all medical examinations at their designated address only. An Examiner *is not permitted* to conduct examinations at a temporary address and is not permitted to name an alternate Examiner. During an Examiner's absence from the permanent office, applicants for airman medical certification shall be referred to another Examiner in the area.

9. Who May Be Certified

a. Age Requirements

There is no age restriction or aviation experience requirement for medical certification. Any applicant who qualifies medically may be issued a Medical Certificate, FAA Form 8500-9 (white), regardless of age. Examiners also have been delegated authority to issue the combined Medical Certificate and Student Pilot Certificate, FAA Form 8420-2 (yellow), which is age restricted because it is an airman medical and student pilot certificate (student license and medical certificate). For issuance of the combined certificate, the applicant must have reached his or her 16th birthday.

Minimum age requirements for the various airman certificates (i.e., pilot license certificates) are defined in 14 CFR part 61, Certification: Pilots and Flight Instructors, and Ground Inspectors as follows:

(1) *Airline transport pilot (ATP) certificate:* 23 years
(2) *Commercial pilot certificate*: 18 years
(3) *Private pilot certificate:* powered aircraft - 17 years;
gliders and balloons - 16 years
(4) *Student pilot certificate:* powered aircraft - 16 years;
gliders and balloons - 14 years

b. Language Requirements

Effective March 5, 2008, the International Civil Aviation Organization (ICAO) (Annex 1 Personnel Licensing) standards require that all Private, Commercial, or Airline Transport pilots as well as Flight Engineers and Flight Navigators operating internationally as required crewmembers of an airplane or helicopter have an airman certificate with an endorsement of language proficiency. In the case of persons holding a U.S. airman certificate, the language proficiency endorsement will state "English Proficient." An applicant for an "Airman Medical and Student Pilot Certificate" must meet the ICAO definition of "English Proficient," which is equivalent to the FAA's long-standing basic English standard.

At each exam, the Examiner must observe the applicant's ability to understand and communicate in English. This may be accomplished by observing the applicant reading instructions, answering questions, and conversing with the AME.

If there is any doubt regarding the applicant's English proficiency:

- Providing Part 67 Medical Qualification Standard is met, applicants for "Airman Medical and Student Pilot Certificate" may be issued the Airman Medical Certificate. **The AME must NOT issue the Student Pilot Certificate.**

- Providing Part 67 Medical Qualification Standard is met, applicants for an Airman Medical Certificate may be issued the Airman Medical Certificate.

- In all cases:

  o The AME must notify the applicant of their concern, *document the notification in block 60,* and advise the applicant to report to the local FSDO for further testing.

  o The AME must also notify the FSDO and or the RFS and *document this in block 60.* If the AME notifies only the RFS, then the RFS must notify the FSDO closest to the examining AME's office. The AME must also *document in block 60 the name of the person contacted.*

The ICAO standard rates individuals from Level 1 (pre-elementary) to Level 6 (expert). Operational Level 4 is considered the minimum for proficiency. The following is provided as information only:

1. PRONUNCIATION
Assumes that English is not the applicant's first language and that the applicant has a dialect or accent that is intelligible to the aeronautical community. Pronunciation, stress, rhythm, and intonation are influenced by the applicant's first language, but only sometimes interfere with ease of understanding.

2. STRUCTURE
Relevant grammatical structures and sentence patterns are determined by language functions appropriate to the task. Basic grammatical structures and sentence patterns are used creatively and are usually well controlled by the applicant. Errors may occur, particularly in unusual or unexpected circumstances, but rarely interfere with meaning.

3. VOCABULARY
The applicant's vocabulary range and accuracy are usually sufficient to communicate effectively on common, concrete, and work-related topics. The applicant can often paraphrase successfully when lacking vocabulary in unusual or unexpected circumstances.

4. FLUENCY

The applicant produces stretches of language at an appropriate tempo. There may be occasional loss of fluency on transition from rehearsed or formulaic speech to spontaneous interaction, but this does not prevent effective communication. The applicant can make limited use of discourse markers or connectors. Fillers are not distracting.

5. COMPREHENSION

Comprehension by the applicant is mostly accurate on common, concrete, and work-related topics when the dialect, accent or variety used is sufficiently intelligible. When the applicant is confronted with a linguistic or situational complication or an unexpected turn of events, comprehension may be slower or require clarification strategies.

6. INTERACTIONS

Responses by the applicant are usually immediate, appropriate, and informative. The applicant initiates and maintains exchanges even when dealing with an unexpected turn of events. The applicant deals adequately with apparent misunderstandings by checking, confirming, or clarifying.

10. Classes of Medical Certificates

An applicant may apply and be granted any class of airman medical certificate as long as the applicant meets the required medical standards for that class of medical certificate. However, an applicant must have the appropriate class of medical certificate for the flying duties the airman intends to exercise. For example, an applicant who exercises the privileges of an airline transport pilot (ATP) certificate must hold a first-class medical certificate. That same pilot when holding only a third-class medical certificate may only exercise privileges of a private pilot certificate. Finally, an applicant need not hold an ATP airman certificate to be eligible for a first-class medical certificate.

Listed below are the three classes of airman medical certificates, identifying the categories of airmen (i.e., pilot) certificates applicable to each class.

First-Class - Airline Transport Pilot

Second-Class - Commercial Pilot; Flight Engineer; Flight Navigator; or Air Traffic Control Tower Operator. (Note: This category of air traffic controller does not include FAA employee air traffic control specialists)

Third-Class - Private Pilot, Recreational Pilot, or Student Pilot

11. Operations Not Requiring a Medical Certificate

Glider and Free Balloon Pilots are not required to hold a medical certificate of any class. To be issued Glider or Free Balloon Airman Certificates, applicants must certify that they do not know, or have reason to know, of any medical condition that would make them unable to operate a glider or free balloon in a safe manner. This certification is made at the local FAA FSDO.

"Sport" pilots are required to hold either a valid airman medical certificate or a current and valid U.S. driver's license. When using a current and valid U.S. driver's license to qualify, sport pilots must comply with each restriction and limitation on their U.S. driver's license and any judicial or administrative order applying to the operation of a motor vehicle.

To exercise sport pilot privileges using a current and valid U.S. driver's license as evidence of qualification sport pilots must:

- Not have been denied the issuance of at least a third-class airman medical certificate (if they have applied for an airman medical certificate)
- Not have had their most recent airman medical certificate revoked or suspended (if they have held an airman medical certificate); and
- Not have had an Authorization withdrawn (if they have ever been granted an Authorization)

Sport pilots may not use a current and valid U.S. driver's license in lieu of a valid airman medical certificate if they know or have reason to know of any medical condition that would make them unable to operate a light-sport aircraft in a safe manner.

Sport pilot medical provisions are found under 14 CFR §§ 61.3, 61.23, 61.53, and 61.303).

For more information about the sport pilot final rule, see the Certification of Aircraft and Airmen for the Operation of Light-Sport Aircraft; Final Rule.

12. Medical Certificates – AME Completion

- Each medical certificate must bear the same date as the date of medical examination regardless of the date the certificate is actually issued.
- Each medical certificate must be type-written either by typewriter or computer print-out. Handwritten or obviously corrected certificates are not acceptable.
- Only use standard limitations as contained within this document or on the Aerospace Medical Certification System (AMCS).
- Each medical certificate must be fully completed prior to being signed.
  - Both the AME and applicant must sign the medical certificate in ink.
  - The applicant must sign before leaving the AME's office.

AMEs are required to use the electronic transmission capability of AMCS and must forward the FAA/Original Copy to the FAA in Oklahoma (see address below). The AME Work Copy must be retained as the file copy.

FAA AEROSPACE MEDICAL CERTIFICATION DIVISION
AAM-300
P.O. Box 26080
OKLAHOMA CITY, OK 73125

13. Validity of Medical Certificates

A. First-Class Medical Certificate: A first-class medical certificate is valid for the remainder of the month of issue; plus

6-calendar months for operations requiring a first-class medical certificate if the airman is age 40 or over on or before the date of the examination, or plus

12-calendar months for operations requiring a first-class medical certificate if the airman has not reached age 40 on or before the date of examination

12-calendar months for operations requiring a second-class medical certificate, or plus

24-calendar months for operations requiring a third-class medical certificate, or plus

60-calendar months for operations requiring a third-class medical certificate if the airman has not reached age 40 on or before the date of examination.

B. Second-Class Medical Certificate: A second-class medical certificate is valid for the remainder of the month of issue; plus

12-calendar months for operations requiring a second-class medical certificate, or plus

24-calendar months for operations requiring a third-class medical certificate, or plus

60-calendar months for operations requiring a third-class medical certificate if the airman has not reached age 40 on or before the date of examination.

C. Third-Class Medical Certificate: A third-class medical certificate is valid for the remainder of the month of issue; plus

24-calendar months for operations requiring a third-class medical certificate, or plus

60-calendar months for operations requiring a third-class medical certificate if the airman has not reached age 40 on or before the date of examination.

Note: Each medical certificate must bear the same date as the date of medical examination regardless of the date the certificate is actually issued. Each medical certificate must be type-written, either by typewriter or computer print-out.

14. Title 14 CFR § 61.53, Prohibition on Operations During Medical Deficiency

NOTE: 14 CFR § 61.53 was revised on July 27, 2004 by adding subparagraph (c)

(a) Operations that require a medical certificate. Except as provided in paragraph (b) of this section, a person who holds a current medical certificate issued under part 67 of this chapter shall not act as pilot in command, or in any other capacity as a required pilot flight crewmember, while that person:

    (1) Knows or has reason to know of any medical condition that would make the person unable to meet the requirements for the medical certificate necessary for the pilot operation; or

    (2) Is taking medication or receiving other treatment for a medical condition that results in the person being unable to meet the requirements for the medical certificate necessary for the pilot operation

(b) Operations that do not require a medical certificate. For operations provided for in § 61.23(b) of this part, a person shall not act as pilot in command, or in any other capacity as a required pilot flight crewmember, while that person knows or has reason to know of any medical condition that would make the person unable to operate the aircraft in a safe manner.

(c) Operations requiring a medical certificate or a U.S. driver's license. For operations provided for in Sec. 61.23(c), a person must meet the provisions of—

    (1) Paragraph (a) of this section if that person holds a valid medical certificate issued under part 67 of this chapter and does not hold a current and valid U.S. driver's license

    (2) Paragraph (b) of this section if that person holds a current and valid U.S. driver's license

15. Reexamination of an Airman

A medical certificate holder may be required to undergo a reexamination at any time if, in the opinion of the Federal Air Surgeon or authorized representative within the FAA, there is a reasonable basis to question the airman's ability to meet the medical standards. An Examiner may **NOT** order such reexamination.

16. Examination Fees

The FAA does not establish fees to be charged by Examiners for the medical examination of persons applying for airman medical certification. It is recommended that the fee be the usual and customary fee established by other physicians in the same general locality for similar services.

17. Replacement of Medical Certificates

Medical certificates that are lost or accidentally destroyed may be replaced upon proper application provided such certificates have not expired. The request should be sent to:

FOIA DESK
AEROSPACE MEDICAL CERTIFICATION DIVISION, AAM-331
FEDERAL AVIATION ADMINISTRATION
CIVIL AEROSPACE MEDICAL INSTITUTE
POST OFFICE BOX 26200
OKLAHOMA CITY, OK 73125-0080

The airman's request for replacement must be accompanied by a remittance of two dollars ($2) (check or money order) made payable to the FAA. This request must include:

- Airman's full name and date of birth;

- Class of certificate;

- Place and date of examination;

- Name of the Examiner; and

- Circumstances of the loss or destruction of the original certificate.

The replacement certificate will be prepared in the same manner as the missing certificate and will bear the same date of examination regardless of when it is issued.

In an emergency, contact your RFS or the Manager, AMCD, AAM-300, at above address or by facsimile at 405-954-4300 for certification verification only.

18. Disposition of Applications and Medical Examinations

All completed applications and medical examinations, except those for student pilots, unless otherwise directed by the FAA, must be transmitted electronically via AMCS within

14 days after completion to the AMCD. **Student pilot examinations must be submitted within 7 days**. These requirements also apply to submissions by International AMEs.

A record of the examination is stored in AMCS, however, Examiners are encouraged to print a copy for their own files. While not required, the Examiner may also print a summary sheet for the applicant.

19. Protection and Destruction of Forms

Forms are available electronically in AMCS. Examiners are accountable for all blank FAA forms they may have printed and are cautioned to provide adequate security for such forms or certificates to ensure that they do not become available for illegal use. Examiners are responsible for destroying any existing paper forms they may still have.

NOTE: Forms should not be shared with other Examiners.

20. Questions or Requests for Assistance

When an Examiner has a question or needs assistance in carrying out responsibilities, the Examiner should contact one of the following individuals:

A. Regional Flight Surgeon (RFS)

- Questions pertaining to problem medical certification cases in which the RFS has initiated action

- Telephone interpretation of medical standards or policies involving an individual airman whom the Examiner is examining

- Matters regarding designation and redesignation of Examiners and the Aviation Medical Examiner Program

- Attendance at Aviation Medical Examiner Seminars

B. Manager, AMCD, AAM-300

- Inquiries concerning guidance on problem medical certification cases

- Information concerning the overall airman medical certification program

- Matters involving FAA medical certification of military personnel

- Information concerning medical certification of applicants in foreign countries

These inquiries should be made to:

MANAGER
AEROSPACE MEDICAL CERTIFICATION DIVISION, AAM-300
CIVIL AEROSPACE MEDICAL INSTITUTE
FEDERAL AVIATION ADMINISTRATION
POST OFFICE BOX 26080
OKLAHOMA CITY, OK 73125

C. Manager, Aeromedical Education Division, AAM-400

- Matters regarding designation and redesignation of Examiners

- Requests for medical forms and stationery

- Requests for airman medical educational material

These inquiries should be made to:

MANAGER
AEROSPACE MEDICAL EDUCATION DIVISION, AAM-400
CIVIL AEROSPACE MEDICAL INSTITUTE
FEDERAL AVIATION ADMINISTRATION
POST OFFICE BOX 26080
OKLAHOMA CITY, OK 73125

21. Airman Appeals

A. Request for Reconsideration

An Examiner's denial of a medical certificate is not a final FAA denial. An applicant may ask for reconsideration of an Examiner's denial by submitting a request in writing to:

FEDERAL AIR SURGEON
ATTN: MANAGER,
AEROSPACE MEDICAL CERTIFICATION DIVISION, AAM-331
CIVIL AEROSPACE MEDICAL INSTITUTE
FEDERAL AVIATION ADMINISTRATION
POST OFFICE BOX 26200
OKLAHOMA CITY, OK 73125-0080

The AMCD will provide initial reconsideration. Some cases may be referred to the appropriate RFS for action. If the AMCD or a RFS finds that the applicant is not qualified, the applicant is denied and advised of further reconsideration and appeal procedures. These may include reconsideration by the Federal Air Surgeon and/or petition for NTSB review.

B. Statement of Demonstrated Ability (SODA)

At the discretion of the Federal Air Surgeon, a Statement of Demonstrated Ability (SODA) may be granted, instead of an Authorization, to a person whose disqualifying condition is static or non-progressive and who has been found capable of performing airman duties without endangering public safety. A SODA does not expire and authorizes a designated Examiner to issue a medical certificate of a specified class if the Examiner finds that the condition described on the SODA has not adversely changed.

In granting a SODA, the Federal Air Surgeon may consider the person's operational experience and any medical facts that may affect the ability of the person to perform airman duties including:

- The combined effect on the person of failure to meet more than one requirement of part 67; and

- The prognosis derived from professional consideration of all available information regarding the person.

In granting a SODA under the special issuance section of part 67 (14 CFR 67.401), the Federal Air Surgeon specifies the class of medical certificate authorized to be issued and may do any of the following:

- State on the SODA, and on any medical certificate based upon it, any operational limitation needed for safety; or

- Condition the continued effect of a SODA, and any second- or third-class medical certificate based upon it, on compliance with a statement of functional limitations issued to the person in coordination with the Director of Flight Standards or the Director's designee

- In determining whether a SODA should be granted to an applicant for a third-class medical certificate, the Federal Air Surgeon considers the freedom of an airman, exercising the privileges of a private pilot certificate, to accept reasonable risks to his or her person and property that are not acceptable in the exercise of commercial or airline transport pilot privileges, and, at the same time, considers the need to protect the safety of persons and property in other aircraft and on the ground

A SODA granted to a person who does not meet the applicable standards of part 67 may be withdrawn, at the discretion of the Federal Air Surgeon, at any time if:

- There is adverse change in the holder's medical condition;

- The holder fails to comply with a statement of functional limitations or operational limitations issued under the special issuance section of part 67 (14 CFR 67.401);

- Public safety would be endangered by the holder's exercise of airman privileges;

- The holder fails to provide medical information reasonably needed by the Federal Air Surgeon for certification under the special issuance section of part 67 (14 CFR 67.401)

- The holder makes or causes to be made a statement or entry that is the basis for withdrawal of a SODA under the falsification section of part 67 (14 CFR 67.403); or

- A person who has been granted a SODA under the special issuance section of part 67 (14 CFR 67.401), based on a special medical flight or practical test need not take the test again during later medical examinations unless the Federal Air Surgeon determines or has reason to believe that the physical deficiency has or may have degraded to a degree to require another special medical flight test or practical test

The authority of the Federal Air Surgeon under the special issuance section of part 67 (14 CFR 67.401) is also exercised by the Manager, AMCD, and each RFS.

If a SODA is withdrawn at any time, the following procedures apply:

- The holder of the SODA will be served a letter of withdrawal stating the reason for the action;

- By not later than 60 days after the service of the letter of withdrawal, the holder of the SODA may request, in writing, that the Federal Air Surgeon provide for review of the decision to withdraw. The request for review may be accompanied by supporting medical evidence;

- Within 60 days of receipt of a request for review, a written final decision either affirming or reversing the decision to withdraw will be issued; and

- A medical certificate rendered invalid pursuant to a withdrawal, in accordance with the special issuance section of part 67 (14 CFR 67.401 (a)) shall be surrendered to the Administrator upon request

C. National Transportation Safety Board (NTSB)

Within 60 days after a final FAA denial of an unrestricted airman medical certificate, an airman may petition the NTSB for a review of that denial. The NTSB does not have jurisdiction to review the denial of a SODA or special issuance airman medical certificate.

A petition for NTSB review must be submitted in writing to:

NATIONAL TRANSPORTATION SAFETY BOARD
490 L'ENFANT PLAZA, EAST SW
WASHINGTON, DC 20594-0001

The NTSB is an independent agency of the Federal Government that has the authority to review on appeal the suspension, amendment, modification, revocation, or denial of any certificate or license issued by the FAA Administrator.

An Administrative Law Judge for the NTSB may hold a formal hearing at which the FAA will present documentary evidence and testimony by medical specialists supporting the denial decision. The petitioner will also be given an opportunity to present evidence and testimony at the hearing. The Administrative Law Judge's decision is subject to review by the full NTSB.

APPLICATION FOR MEDICAL CERTIFICATION

Items 1-20 of FAA Form 8500-8

ITEMS 1- 20 of FAA Form 8500-8

This section contains guidance for items on the Medical History and General Information page of FAA Form 8500-8, Application for Airman Medical Certificate or Airman Medical and Student Pilot Certificate.

I. AME Guidance for Positive Identification of Airmen and Application Procedures

All applicants must show proof of age and identity under 14 CFR §67.4. On occasion, individuals have attempted to be examined under a false name. If the applicant is unknown to the Examiner, the Examiner should request evidence of positive identification. A Government-issued photo identification (e.g., driver's license, identification card issued by a driver's license authority, military identification, or passport) provides age and identity and is preferred. Applicants may use other government-issued identification for age (e.g., certified copy of a birth certificate); however, the Examiner must request separate photo identification for identity (such as a work badge). Verify that the address provided is the same as that given under Item 5. Record the type of identification(s) provided and identifying number(s) under Item 61. Make a copy of the identification and keep it on file for 3 years with the AME work copy.

An applicant who does not have government-issued photo identification may use non-photo government-issued identification (e.g. pilot certificate, birth certificate, voter registration card) in conjunction with a photo identification (e.g. work identification card, student identification card).

If an airman fails to provide identification, the Examiner must report this immediately to the AMCD, or the appropriate RFS for guidance.

II. Prior to the Examination

- Once the applicant successfully completes Items 1-20 of FAA Form 8500-8 through the FAA MedXPress (MedX) system, he/she will receive a confirmation number and instructions to print a summary sheet. **This data entered through the MedXPress system will remain valid for 60 days.**

- Applicants must bring their MedX confirmation number, valid photo identification, and the summary sheet to the Exam. If the applicant does not bring their confirmation number to the exam, the applicant can retrieve it from MedX or their email account. Examiners should call AMCS Support if the confirmation number cannot be retrieved.

- Examiners **must not** begin the exam until they have imported the MedX application into AMCS and have verified the identity of the applicant.

III. After the Applicant Completes the Medical History of the FAA Form 8500-8

The Examiner must review all Items 1 through 20 for accuracy. The applicant must answer all questions. The date for Item 16 may be estimated if the applicant does not recall the actual date of the last examination. However, for the sake of electronic transmission, it must be placed in the mm/dd/yyyy format.

Verify that the name on the applicant's identification media matches the name on the FAA Form 8500-8. If it does not, question the applicant for an explanation. If the explanation is not reasonable (legal name change, subsequent marriage, etc.), do not continue the medical examination or issue a medical certificate. Contact your RFS for guidance.

The applicant's Social Security Number (SSN) is not mandatory. Failure to provide is not grounds for refusal to issue a medical certificate. (See **Item 4**). All other items on the form must be completed.

Applicants must provide their home address on the FAA Form 8500-8. Applicants may use a private mailing address (e.g., a P.O. Box number or a mail drop) if that is their preferred mailing address; however, under Item 18 (in the "Explanations" box) of the FAA Form 8500-8, they must provide their home address.

An applicant cannot make updates to their application once they have certified and submitted it. If the examiner discovers the need for corrections to the application during the review, the Examiner is required to discuss these changes with the applicant and obtain their approval. The examiner must make any changes to the application in AMCS.

Strict compliance with this procedure is essential in case it becomes necessary for the FAA to take legal action for falsification of the application.

ITEMS 1-2. Application for; Class of Medical Certificate Applied For

The applicant indicates whether the application is for an Airman Medical Certificate (white) or an Airman Medical and Student Pilot Certificate (yellow), and the class of medical certificate desired.

The class of medical certificate sought by the applicant is needed so that the appropriate medical standards may be applied. The class of certificate issued must correspond with that for which the applicant has applied.

The applicant may ask for a medical certificate of a higher class than needed for the type of flying or duties currently performed. For example, a student pilot may ask for a first-class medical certificate to see if he or she qualifies medically before entry into an aviation career.

The Examiner applies the standards appropriate to the class sought, not to the airman's duties - either performed or anticipated. The Examiner should never issue more than one certificate based on the same examination.

ITEMS 3-10. Identification

Items 3-10 on the FAA Form 8500-8 must be entered as identification. While most of the items are self-explanatory (as indicated in the MedXPress drop-down menu next to individual items) specific instructions include:

- **Item 3. Last Name; First Name; Middle Name**
  The applicant's legal last, first, and middle name (or initial if appropriate) must be provided.

- **Item 4. Social Security Number (SSN)**
  The applicant must provide their SSN. If they decline to provide one or are an international applicant, they must check the appropriate box and a number will be generated for them. The FAA requests a SSN for identification purposes, record control, and to prevent mistakes in identification.

- **Item 6. Date of Birth**
  The applicant **must** enter the numbers for the month, day, and year of birth in order. Name, date of birth, and SSN are the basic identifiers of airmen. When an Examiner communicates with the FAA concerning an applicant, the Examiner must give the applicant's full name, date of birth, and SSN if at all possible. The applicant should indicate citizenship; e.g., U.S.A.

If the applicant is seeking an Airman Medical and Student Pilot Certificate (FAA Form 8420-2), the Examiner should check the date of birth to ensure that the applicant is at least 16 years old. Unless the applicant is at least 16 years old, a combined Airman Medical and Student Pilot Certificate may not be issued, even if the applicant will become 16 years old before the certificate expires (except as noted below).

The FAA **will not confirm** a certificate issued by an Examiner to a person who is less than 16 years old. The applicant must be at least 16 years old **at the time of application** to be eligible for a student pilot certificate for flight of powered aircraft. This minimum age requirement applies only to the issuance of the yellow FAA Form 8420-2, and never to the issuance of the white medical certificate (FAA Form 8500-9).

If the applicant is not yet 16 years old and wishes to solo on or after his or her 16th birthday, the Examiner should issue a white FAA Form 8500-9 (if the applicant is fully qualified medically). On or after his or her 16th birthday, the applicant may obtain a student pilot certificate for the flight from a FAA Flight Standards District Office (FSDO) or designated Flight Examiner upon presentation of the FAA Form 8500-9 (white medical certificate).

An alternative procedure for this situation is for the Examiner to issue the Airman Medical and Student Pilot Certificate, FAA Form 8420-2 (yellow), with the following statement in the limitations block of the student pilot certificate:

NOT VALID UNTIL (MONTH, DAY, AND YEAR OF 16TH BIRTHDAY)

This procedure should not be used if the applicant's 16th birthday will occur more than 30 days from the date of application.

Although nonmedical regulations allow an airman to solo a glider or balloon at age 14, a medical certificate is not required for glider or balloon operations. These airmen are required to certify to the FAA that they have no known physical defects that make them unable to pilot a glider or balloon. This certification is made at the FAA FSDO's.

There is a maximum age requirement for certain air carrier pilots. Because this is not a medical requirement but an operational one, the Examiner may issue medical certificates without regard to age to any applicant who meets the medical standards.

ITEMS 11-12. Occupation; Employer

Occupational data are principally used for statistical purposes. This information, along with information obtained from **Items 10, 14** and **15** may be important in determining whether a SODA may be issued, if applicable.

11. Occupation

This should reflect the applicant's major employment. "Pilot" should only be reported when the applicant earns a livelihood from flying.

12. Employer

The employer's name should be entered by the applicant.

ITEM 13. Has Your FAA Airman Medical Certificate Ever Been Denied, Suspended, or Revoked?

The applicant shall check "yes" or "no." If "yes" is checked, the applicant should enter the date of action and should report details in the EXPLANATIONS box of **Item 18**.

The Examiner may not issue a medical certificate to an applicant who has checked "yes." The only exceptions to this prohibition are:

- The applicant presents written evidence from the FAA that he or she was subsequently medically certificated and that an Examiner is authorized to issue a renewal medical certificate to the person if medically qualified; or

- The Examiner obtains oral or written authorization to issue a medical certificate from an FAA medical office

ITEMS 14-15. Total Pilot Time

14. Total Pilot Time to Date

The applicant should indicate the total number of *civilian* flight hours and whether those hours are logged (LOG) or estimated (EST).

15. Total Pilot Time Past 6 Months

The applicant should provide the number of *civilian* flight hours in the 6-month period immediately preceding the date of this application. The applicant should indicate whether those hours are logged (LOG) or estimated (EST).

ITEM 16. Date of Last FAA Medical Application

If a prior application was made, the applicant should indicate the date of the last application, even if it is only an estimate of the year. This item should be completed even if the application was made many years ago or the previous application *did not result in the issuance* of a medical certificate. If no prior application was made, the applicant should check the appropriate block in Item 16.

ITEM 17.a. Do You Currently Use Any Medication (Prescription or NONprescription)?

If the applicant checks yes, give name of medication(s) and indicate if the medication was listed in a previous FAA medical examination.

This includes both prescription and nonprescription medication. (Additional guidelines for the certification of airmen who use medication may be found in throughout the Guide).

For example, any airman who is undergoing continuous treatment with anticoagulants, antiviral agents, anxiolytics, barbiturates, chemotherapeutic agents, experimental hypoglycemic, investigational, mood-ameliorating, motion sickness, narcotic, sedating antihistaminic, sedative, steroid drugs, or tranquilizers must be deferred certification *unless* the treatment has previously been cleared by FAA medical authority. In such an instance, the applicant should provide the Examiner with a copy of any FAA correspondence that supports the clearance.

During periods in which the foregoing medications are being used for treatment of acute illnesses, the airman is under obligation to refrain from exercising the privileges of his/her airman medical certificate unless cleared by the FAA.

Further information concerning an applicant's use of medication may be found under the items pertaining to specific medical condition(s) for which the medication is used, or you may contact your RFS.

ITEM 17.b. Do You Ever Use Near Vision Contact Lens(es) While Flying?

The applicant should indicate whether near vision contact lens(es) is/are used while flying. If the applicant answers "yes," the Examiner must counsel the applicant that **use of contact lens(es) for monovision correction is not allowed.** The Examiner must note in Item 60 that this counseling has been given. **Examples of unacceptable use include:**

- The use of a contact lens in one eye for near vision and in the other eye for distant vision (for example: pilots with myopia plus presbyopia).

- The use of a contact lens in one eye for near vision and the use of no contact lens in the other eye (for example: pilots with presbyopia but no myopia).

If the applicant checks "yes" and no further comment is noted on FAA Form 8500-8 by either the applicant or the Examiner, a letter will automatically be sent to the applicant informing him or her that such use is/are inappropriate for flying.

Please note: the use of **binocular** contact lenses for distance-correction-only is acceptable. In this instance, no special evaluation or SODA is routinely required for a distance-vision-only contact lens wearer who meets the standard and has no complications. **Binocular** bifocal or binocular multifocal contact lenses are also acceptable under the Protocol for Binocular Multifocal and Accommodating Devices. If the applicant checks "yes" in Item 17.b but actually is using **binocular** bifocal or binocular multifocal contact lenses then the Examiner should note this in **Item 60.**

ITEM 18. Medical History

Each item under this heading must be checked either "yes" or "no." For all items checked "yes," a description and approximate date of every condition the applicant has ever been diagnosed with, had, or presently has, must be given in the EXPLANATIONS box. If information has been reported on a previous application for airman medical certification and there has been no change in the condition, the applicant may note "PREVIOUSLY REPORTED, NO CHANGE" in the EXPLANATIONS box, but the applicant must still check "yes" to the condition.

Of particular importance are conditions that have developed since the last FAA medical examination. The Examiner must take the time to review the applicant's responses on FAA Form 8500-8 before starting the applicant's medical examination.

The Examiner should ensure that the applicant has checked all of the boxes in Item 18 as either "yes" or "no." The Examiner should use information obtained from this review in asking the applicant pertinent questions during the course of the examination.

Certain aspects of the individual's history may need to be elaborated upon. The Examiner should provide in Item 60 an explanation of the nature of items checked "yes" in items 18.a. through 18.y. Please be aware there is a character count limit in Item 60. If all comments cannot fit in Item 60, the Examiner may submit additional information on a plain sheet of paper and include the applicant's full name, date of birth, signature, any appropriate identifying numbers (PI, MID or SSN), and the date of the exam.

Supplementary reports from the applicant's physician(s) should be obtained and forwarded to the AMCD, when necessary, to clarify the significance of an item of history. The responsibility for providing such supplementary reports rests with the applicant. A discussion with the Examiner's RFS may clarify and expedite the certification process at that time.

Affirmative answers alone in Item 18 do not constitute a basis for denial of a medical certificate. A decision concerning issuance or denial should be made by applying the medical standards pertinent to the conditions uncovered by the history.

Experience has shown that, when asked direct questions by a physician, applicants are likely to be candid and willing to discuss medical problems.

The Examiner should attempt to establish rapport with the applicant and to develop a complete medical history. Further, the Examiner should be familiar with the FAA certification policies and procedures in order to provide the applicant with sound advice.

18.a. Frequent or severe headaches. The applicant should report frequency, duration, characteristics, severity of symptoms, neurologic manifestations, and whether they have been incapacitating, treatment and side effects, if any. (See **Item 46**)

18.b. Dizziness or fainting spells. The applicant should describe characteristics of the episode; e.g., spinning or lightheadedness, frequency, factors leading up to and surrounding the episode, associated neurologic symptoms; e.g., headache, nausea, LOC, or paresthesias. Include diagnostic workup and treatment if any.
(See **Items 25-30** and **Item 46**)

18.c. Unconsciousness for any reason. The applicant should describe the event(s) to determine the primary organ system responsible for the episode, witness statements, initial treatment, and evidence of recurrence or prior episode. Although the regulation states, "an unexplained disturbance of consciousness is disqualifying," it does not mean to imply that the applicant can be certificated if the etiology is identified, because the etiology may also be disqualifying in and of itself. (See **Item 46**).

18.d. Eye or vision trouble except glasses. The Examiner should personally explore the applicant's history by asking questions, concerning any changes in vision, unusual visual experiences (halos, scintillations, etc.), sensitivity to light, injuries, surgery, or current use of medication. Does the applicant report inordinate difficulties with eye fatigue or strain? Is there a history of serious eye disease such as glaucoma or other disease commonly associated with secondary eye changes, such as diabetes? For glaucoma or ocular hypertension, obtain a FAA Form 8500-14, Report of Eye Evaluation for Glaucoma. For any other medical condition, obtain a FAA Form 8500-7, Report of Eye Evaluation. Under all circumstances, please advise the examining eye specialist to explain why the airman is unable to correct to Snellen visual acuity of 20/20. (See **Items 31-34, Item 53,** and **Item 54**)

18.e. Hay fever or allergy. The applicant should report frequency and duration of symptoms, any incapacitation by the condition, treatment, and side effects. The Examiner should inquire whether the applicant has ever experienced any barotitis ("ear block"), barosinusitis, alternobaric vertigo, or any other symptoms that could interfere with aviation safety. (See **Item 26**)

18.f. Asthma or lung disease. The applicant should provide frequency and severity of asthma attacks, medications, and number of visits to the hospital and/or emergency room. For other lung conditions, a detailed description of symptoms/diagnosis, surgical intervention, and medications should be provided. (See **Item 35**)

18.g. Heart or vascular trouble. The applicant should describe the condition to include, dates, symptoms, and treatment, and provide medical reports to assist in the certification decision-making process. These reports should include: operative reports of coronary intervention to include the original cardiac catheterization report, stress tests, worksheets, and original tracings (or a legible copy). When stress tests are provided, forward the reports, worksheets and original tracings (or a legible copy) to the FAA. Part 67 provides that, for all classes of medical certificates, an established medical history or clinical diagnosis of myocardial infarction, angina pectoris, cardiac valve replacement, permanent cardiac pacemaker implantation, heart replacement, or coronary heart disease that has required treatment or, if untreated, that has been symptomatic or clinically significant, is cause for denial. (See **Item 36**)

18.h. High or low blood pressure. The applicant should provide history and treatment. Issuance of a medical certificate to an applicant with high blood pressure may depend on the current blood pressure levels and whether the applicant is taking anti-hypertensive medication. The Examiner should also determine if the applicant has a history of complications, adverse reactions to therapy, hospitalization, etc. (Details are given in **Item 36** and **Item 55**).

18.i. Stomach, liver, or intestinal trouble. The applicant should provide history and treatment, pertinent medical records, current status report, and medication. If a surgical procedure was done, the applicant must provide operative and pathology reports. (See **Item 38**).

18.j. Kidney stone or blood in urine. The applicant should provide history and treatment, pertinent medical records, current status report and medication. If a procedure was done, the applicant must provide the report and pathology reports. (See **Item 41**).

18.k. Diabetes. The applicant should describe the condition to include, symptoms and treatment. Comment on the presence or absence of hyperglycemic and/or hypoglycemic episodes. A medical history or clinical diagnosis of diabetes mellitus requiring insulin or other hypoglycemic drugs for control are disqualifying. The Examiner can help expedite the FAA review by assisting the applicant in gathering medical records and submitting a current specialty report. (See **Item 48**)

18.l. Neurological disorders; epilepsy, seizures, stroke, paralysis, etc. The applicant should provide history and treatment, pertinent medical records, current status report and medication. The Examiner should obtain details about such a history and report the results. An established diagnosis of epilepsy, a transient loss of control of nervous system function(s), or a disturbance of consciousness is a basis for denial no matter how remote the history. Like all other conditions of aeromedical concern, the history surrounding the event is crucial. Certification is possible if a satisfactory explanation can be established. (See **Item 46**)

18.m. Mental disorders of any sort; depression, anxiety, etc. An affirmative answer to Item 18.m. requires investigation through supplemental history taking. Dispositions will vary according to the details obtained. An applicant with an established history of a personality disorder that is severe enough to have repeatedly manifested itself by overt acts, a psychosis disorder, or a bipolar disorder must be denied or deferred by the Examiner. (See **Item 47**)

18.n. Substance dependence; or failed a drug test ever; or substance abuse or use of illegal substance in the last 2 years. "Substance" includes alcohol and other drugs (e.g., PCP, sedatives and hypnotics, anxiolytics, marijuana, cocaine, opioids, amphetamines, hallucinogens, and other psychoactive drugs or chemicals). For a "yes" answer to Item 18.n., the Examiner should obtain a detailed description of the history. A history of substance dependence or abuse is disqualifying. The Examiner must defer issuance of a certificate if there is doubt concerning an applicant's substance use. (See **Item 47**)

18.o. Alcohol dependence or abuse. (See Item **18.n.**)

18.p. Suicide attempt. A history of suicidal attempts or suicidal gestures requires further evaluation. The ultimate decision of whether an applicant with such a history is eligible for medical certification rests with the FAA. The Examiner should take a supplemental history as indicated, assist in the gathering of medical records related to the incident(s), and, if the applicant agrees, assist in obtaining psychiatric and/or psychological examinations. (See **Item 47**)

18.q. Motion sickness requiring medication. A careful history concerning the nature of the sickness, frequency and need for medication is indicated when the applicant responds affirmatively to this item. Because motion sickness varies with the nature of the stimulus, it is most helpful to know if the problem has occurred in flight or under similar circumstances. (See **Item 29**)

18.r. Military medical discharge. If the person has received a military medical discharge, the Examiner should take additional history and record it in **Item 60**. It is helpful to know the circumstances surrounding the discharge, including dates, and whether the individual is receiving disability compensation. If the applicant is receiving veteran's disability benefits, the claim number and service number are helpful in obtaining copies of pertinent medical records. The fact that the applicant is receiving disability benefits does not necessarily mean that the application should be denied.

18.s. Medical rejection by military service. The Examiner should inquire about the place, cause, and date of rejection and enter the information in **Item 60**. It is helpful if the Examiner can assist the applicant with obtaining relevant military documents. If a delay of more than 14-calendar days is expected, the Examiner should transmit FAA Form 8500-8 to the FAA with a note specifying what documents will be forwarded later.

Disposition will depend upon whether the medical condition still exists or whether a history of such a condition requires denial or deferral under the FAA medical standards.

18.t. Rejection for life or health insurance. The Examiner should inquire regarding the circumstances of rejection. The supplemental history should be recorded in **Item 60**. Disposition will depend upon whether the medical condition still exists or whether a history of such a condition requires denial or deferral under the FAA medical standards.

18.u. Admission to hospital. For each admission, the applicant should list the dates, diagnoses, duration, treatment, name of the attending physician, and complete address of the hospital or clinic. If previously reported, the applicant may enter "PREVIOUSLY REPORTED, NO CHANGE." A history of hospitalization does not disqualify an applicant, although the medical condition that resulted in hospitalization may.

18.v. History of Arrest(s), Conviction(s), and/or Administrative Action(s).
Arrest(s), conviction(s) and/or administrative action(s) affecting driving privileges may raise questions about the applicant's fitness for certification and may be cause for disqualification. (See Items 18.n. and 47). A single driving while intoxicated (DWI) arrest, conviction and/or administrative action usually is not cause for denial provided there are no other instances or indications of substance dependence or abuse.

The events to be reported are specifically identified in Item 18.v. of FAA Form 8500-8. If **yes** is checked, the applicant must describe the arrest(s), conviction(s), and/or administrative action(s) in the EXPLANATIONS box. The description must include:

- The alcohol or drug offense for which the applicant was arrested, convicted, or the type of administrative action involved (e.g., attendance at an educational or rehabilitation program in lieu of conviction; license denial, suspension, cancellation, or revocation for refusal to be tested; educational safe driving program for multiple speeding convictions; etc.);
- The name of the state or other jurisdiction involved; and
- The date of the arrest, conviction, and/or administrative action

Note: If the applicant documented ALL of the above information on previous exams AND there are no new arrest(s), conviction(s), and/or administrative action(s) since the last application, the applicant may enter **PREVIOUSLY REPORTED, NO CHANGE**.

For all first-time reports of arrest(s), conviction(s), and/or administrative action(s) the Examiner must do the following prior to issuing an airman medical certificate:

- Obtain a detailed history of the applicant's alcohol use, the circumstances surrounding **all** alcohol-related incidents (include those reported in 18v and any others that may have occurred)
- Obtain copies of all court records and arrest reports related to the event(s) **if the incident(s) occurred within the 5 years prior to the exam.** This includes copies of relevant military records if the incidents occurred while the applicant was a member of the U.S. armed forces (includes military court records, records of non-judicial punishment, and military substance abuse records)
- Document those findings in Item 60. (See Item 47)
- Forward the court records, arrest reports, and any military records to AMCD
- Advise the applicant that the reporting of alcohol or drug offenses (i.e., motor vehicle violation) on the history part of the medical application does not relieve the airman of responsibility to report each motor vehicle action to the FAA within 60 days of the occurrence to the:

Security and Investigations Division
AMC-700
P.O. Box 25810
Oklahoma City, OK 73125-0810

Deferral Criteria: The Examiner must defer certification for any of the following:

- Inability to obtain and review the court and arrest records within 14 days of the date of the exam
- For the alcohol- or drug-related driving incidents:
  - Any arrest, conviction, and/or administrative action for which the applicant registers a blood alcohol level 0.15 or higher
  - Any arrest, conviction, and/or administrative action for which the applicant refused blood alcohol testing

- o Any arrest, conviction, and/or administrative action within the preceding 2 years AND THERE HAS BEEN ANOTHER arrest, conviction and/or administrative action AT ANY OTHER TIME
- o Total of 3 arrest(s), conviction(s), and/or administrative action(s) within a lifetime
- o Total of 2 arrest(s), conviction(s), and/or administrative action(s) within the preceding 10 years

If the applicant is deferred, the FAA will require the applicant to:

Provide:
- A detailed personal statement regarding his/her past and present patterns of alcohol or drug use
- A complete copy of his/her current driving record in any state that he/she has held a driver's license in the last 10 years
- Copies of any court records and arrest reports related to the event(s) that have not already been provided to the AME. This includes copies of relevant military records if any event(s) occurred while the applicant was a member of the U.S. armed forces. "Relevant military records" means military court records, records of non-judicial punishment, and military substance abuse records

Obtain:
- A substance abuse evaluation from an addictionologist or addiction psychologist/psychiatrist familiar with aviation standards

Issue Criteria: The Examiner may issue if:

- **NONE of the Deferral Criteria above are met**
- **For reported incident(s) when the most recent incident occurred more than 5 years prior to the exam**, based on the exam and a detailed interview, the Examiner determines the applicant's history does not indicate a possible substance abuse or dependence problem
- **For reported incident(s) when the most recent incident occurred within the preceding 5 years of the exam**, based on the exam, detailed interview **AND** review of the court record(s) and arrest report(s), the Examiner determines the applicant's history does not indicate a possible substance abuse or dependence problem

For guidance on indicators of substance abuse or dependence see:
- o Aerospace Medical Dispositions, Item 47 – Substance Abuse
- o Aerospace Medical Dispositions, Item 47 – Substance Dependence

18.w. History of nontraffic convictions. The applicant must report any other (nontraffic) convictions (e.g., assault, battery, public intoxication, robbery, etc.). The applicant must name the charge for which convicted and the date of the conviction(s), and copies of court documents (if available). (See **Item 47**)

18.x. Other illness, disability, or surgery. The applicant should describe the nature of these illnesses in the EXPLANATIONS box. If additional records, tests, or specialty reports are necessary in order to make a certification decision, the applicant should so be advised. If the applicant does not wish to provide the information requested by the Examiner, the Examiner should defer issuance.

If the applicant wishes to have the FAA review the application and decide what ancillary documentation is needed, the Examiner should defer issuance of the medical certificate and forward the completed FAA Form 8500-8 to the AMCD. If the Examiner proceeds to obtain documentation, but all data will not be received with the 2 weeks, FAA Form 8500-8 should be transmitted immediately to the AMCD with a note that additional documents will be forwarded later under separate cover.

18. y. Medical Disability Benefits. The applicant must report any disability benefits received, regardless of source or amount. If the applicant checks "yes" on this item, the FAA may verify with other Federal Agencies (ie. Social Security Administration, Veteran's Affairs) whether the applicant is receiving a disability benefit that may present a conflict in issuing an FAA medical certificate. The Examiner must document the specifics and nature of the disability in findings in **Item 60**.

ITEM 19. Visits to Health Professional Within Last 3 Years

The applicant should list all visits in the last 3 years to a physician, physician assistant, nurse practitioner, psychologist, clinical social worker, or substance abuse specialist for treatment, examination, or medical/mental evaluation. The applicant should list visits for counseling only if related to a personal substance abuse or psychiatric condition. The applicant should give the name, date, address, and type of health professional consulted and briefly state the reason for the consultation. Multiple visits to one health professional for the same condition may be aggregated on one line.

Routine dental, eye, and FAA periodic medical examinations and consultations with an employer-sponsored employee assistance program (EAP) may be excluded unless the consultations were for the applicant's substance abuse or unless the consultations resulted in referral for psychiatric evaluation or treatment.

When an applicant does provide history in Item 19, the Examiner should review the matter with the applicant. The Examiner will record in **Item 60** only that information needed to document the review and provide the basis for a certification decision. If the Examiner finds the information to be of a personal or sensitive nature with no relevancy to flying safety, it should be recorded in **Item 60** as follows:

"Item 19. Reviewed with applicant. History not significant or relevant to application."

If the applicant is otherwise qualified, a medical certificate may be issued by the Examiner.

FAA medical authorities, upon review of the application, will ask for further information regarding visits to health care providers only where the physical findings, report of examination, applicant disclosure, or other evidence suggests the possible presence of a disqualifying medical history or condition.

If an explanation has been given on a previous report(s) and there has been no change in the condition, the applicant may enter "PREVIOUSLY REPORTED, NO CHANGE."

Of particular importance is the reporting of conditions that have developed since the applicant's last FAA medical examination. The Examiner is asked to comment on all entries, including those "PREVIOUSLY REPORTED, NO CHANGE." These comments may be entered under **Item 60**.

ITEM 20. Applicant's National Driver Register and Certifying Declaration

In addition to making a declaration of the completeness and truthfulness of the applicant's responses on the medical application, the applicant's declaration authorizes the National Driver Register to release the applicant's adverse driving history information, if any, to the FAA. The FAA uses such information to verify information provided in the application. Applicant must certify the declaration outlined in Item 20. If the applicant does not certify the declaration for any reason, Examiner shall not issue a medical certificate but forward the incomplete application to the AMCD.

EXAMINATION TECHNIQUES AND CRITERIA FOR QUALIFICATION

Items 21-58 of FAA Form 8500-8

ITEMS 21- 58 of FAA Form 8500-8

The Examiner must personally conduct the physical examination. This section provides guidance for completion of Items 21-58 of the Application for Airman Medical Certificate or Airman Medical and Student Pilot Certificate, FAA Form 8500-8.

The Examiner must carefully read the applicant's history page of FAA Form 8500-8 (Items 1-20) *before* conducting the physical examination and completing the Report of Medical Examination. This alerts the Examiner to possible pathological findings.

The Examiner must note in **Item 60** of the FAA Form 8500-8 any condition found in the course of the examination. The Examiner must list the facts, such as dates, frequency, and severity of occurrence.

When a question arises, the Federal Air Surgeon encourages Examiners first to check this Guide for Aviation Medical Examiners and other FAA informational documents. If the question remains unresolved, the Examiner should seek advice from a RFS or the Manager of the AMCD.

ITEMS 21-22. Height and Weight

21. Height (inches)	22. Weight (pounds)

ITEM 21. Height

Measure and record the applicant's height in inches. Although there are no medical standards for height, exceptionally short individuals may not be able to effectively reach all flight controls and must fly specially modified aircraft. If required, the FAA will place operational limitations on the pilot certificate.

ITEM 22. Weight

Measure and record the applicant's weight in pounds.

BMI CHART AND FORMULA TABLE

Measurement Units	BMI Formula and Calculation
Pounds and inches	Formula: weight (lb) / [height (in)]^2 x 703 Calculate BMI by dividing weight in pounds (lbs) by height in inches (in) squared and multiplying by a conversion factor of 703. Example: Weight = 150 lbs, Height = 5'5" (65") Calculation: [150 ÷ (65)^2] x 703 = 24.96
Kilograms and meters (or centimeters)	Formula: weight (kg) / [height (m)]2 With the metric system, the formula for BMI is weight in kilograms divided by height in meters squared. Since height is commonly measured in centimeters, divide height in centimeters by 100 to obtain height in meters. Example: Weight = 68 kg, Height = 165 cm (1.65 m) Calculation: 68 ÷ (1.65)2 = 24.98

Body Mass Index Table

	Normal						Overweight					Obese									Extreme Obesity															
BMI	19	20	21	22	23	24	25	26	27	28	29	30	31	32	33	34	35	36	37	38	39	40	41	42	43	44	45	46	47	48	49	50	51	52	53	54
Height (inches)													Body Weight (pounds)																							
58	91	96	100	105	110	115	119	124	129	134	138	143	148	153	158	162	167	172	177	181	186	191	196	201	205	210	215	220	224	229	234	239	244	248	253	258
59	94	99	104	109	114	119	124	128	133	138	143	148	153	158	163	168	173	178	183	188	193	198	203	208	212	217	222	227	232	237	242	247	252	257	262	267
60	97	102	107	112	118	123	128	133	138	143	148	153	158	163	168	174	179	184	189	194	199	204	209	215	220	225	230	235	240	245	250	255	261	266	271	276
61	100	106	111	116	122	127	132	137	143	148	153	158	164	169	174	180	185	190	195	201	206	211	217	222	227	232	238	243	248	254	259	264	269	275	280	285
62	104	109	115	120	126	131	136	142	147	153	158	164	169	175	180	186	191	196	202	207	213	218	224	229	235	240	246	251	256	262	267	273	278	284	289	295
63	107	113	118	124	130	135	141	146	152	158	163	169	175	180	186	191	197	203	208	214	220	225	231	237	242	248	254	259	265	270	278	282	287	293	299	304
64	110	116	122	128	134	140	145	151	157	163	169	174	180	186	192	197	204	209	215	221	227	232	238	244	250	256	262	267	273	279	285	291	296	302	308	314
65	114	120	126	132	138	144	150	156	162	168	174	180	186	192	198	204	210	216	222	228	234	240	246	252	258	264	270	276	282	288	294	300	306	312	318	324
66	118	124	130	136	142	148	155	161	167	173	179	186	192	198	204	210	216	223	229	235	241	247	253	260	266	272	278	284	291	297	303	309	315	322	328	334
67	121	127	134	140	146	153	159	166	172	178	185	191	198	204	211	217	223	230	236	242	249	255	261	268	274	280	287	293	299	306	312	319	325	331	338	344
68	125	131	138	144	151	158	164	171	177	184	190	197	203	210	216	223	230	236	243	249	256	262	269	276	282	289	295	302	308	315	322	328	335	341	348	354
69	128	135	142	149	155	162	169	176	182	189	196	203	209	216	223	230	236	243	250	257	263	270	277	284	291	297	304	311	318	324	331	338	345	351	358	365
70	132	139	146	153	160	167	174	181	188	195	202	209	216	222	229	236	243	250	257	264	271	278	285	292	299	306	313	320	327	334	341	348	355	362	369	376
71	136	143	150	157	165	172	179	186	193	200	208	215	222	229	236	243	250	257	265	272	279	286	293	301	308	315	322	329	338	343	351	358	365	372	379	386
72	140	147	154	162	169	177	184	191	199	206	213	221	228	235	242	250	258	265	272	279	287	294	302	309	316	324	331	338	346	353	361	368	375	383	390	397
73	144	151	159	166	174	182	189	197	204	212	219	227	235	242	250	257	265	272	280	288	295	302	310	318	325	333	340	348	355	363	371	378	386	393	401	408
74	148	155	163	171	179	186	194	202	210	218	225	233	241	249	256	264	272	280	287	295	303	311	319	326	334	342	350	358	365	373	381	389	396	404	412	420
75	152	160	168	176	184	192	200	208	216	224	232	240	248	256	264	272	279	287	295	303	311	319	327	335	343	351	359	367	375	383	391	399	407	415	423	431
76	156	164	172	180	189	197	205	213	221	230	238	246	254	263	271	279	287	295	304	312	320	328	336	344	353	361	369	377	385	394	402	410	418	426	435	443

Source: Adapted from Clinical Guidelines on the Identification, Evaluation, and Treatment of Overweight and Obesity in Adults: The Evidence Report.

ITEMS 23-24. Statement of Demonstrated Ability (SODA); SODA Serial Number

23. Statement of Demonstrated Ability (SODA)	
☐ Yes ☐ No	Defect Noted:

ITEM 23. Has a SODA ever been issued?

Ask the applicant if a SODA has ever been issued. If the answer is "yes," ask the applicant to show you the document. Then check the "yes" block and record the nature and degree of the defect.

SODA's are valid for an indefinite period or until an adverse change occurs that results in a level of defect worse than that stated on the face of the document.

The FAA issues SODA's for certain static defects, but not for disqualifying condition or conditions that may be progressive. The extent of the functional loss that has been cleared by the FAA is stated on the face of the SODA. If the Examiner finds the condition has become worse, a medical certificate should not be issued even if the applicant is otherwise qualified. The Examiner should also defer issuance if it is unclear whether the applicant's present status represents an adverse change.

The Examiner must take special care not to issue a medical certificate of a higher class than that specified on the face of the SODA even if the applicant appears to be otherwise medically qualified. The Examiner may note in **Item 60** the applicant's desire for a higher class.

ITEM 24. SODA Serial Number

24. SODA Serial Number

Enter the assigned serial number in the space provided.

ITEMS 25-30. Ear, Nose and Throat (ENT)

CHECK EACH ITEM IN APPROPRIATE COLUMN	Normal	Abnormal
25. Head, face, neck, and scalp		
26. Nose		
27. Sinuses		
28. Mouth and Throat		
29. Ears, general (internal and external canals: Hearing under Item 49)		
30. Ear Drums (Perforation)		

I. Code of Federal Regulations

All Classes: 14 CFR 67.105(b)(c), 67.205(b)(c), and 67.305(b)(c)

(b) No disease or condition of the middle or internal ear, nose, oral cavity,   pharynx, or larynx that -

(1) Interferes with, or is aggravated by, flying or may reasonably be expected to do so; or

(2) Interferes with, or may reasonably be expected to interfere with, clear and effective speech communication.

(c) No disease or condition manifested by, or that may reasonably be expected to be manifested by, vertigo or a disturbance of equilibrium.

II. Examination Techniques

1. The *head and neck* should be examined to determine the presence of any significant defects such as:

    a. Bony defects of the skull
    b. Gross deformities
    c. Fistulas
    d. Evidence of recent blows or trauma to the head
    e. Limited motion of the head and neck
    f. Surgical scars

2. The *external ear* is seldom a major problem in the medical certification of applicants. Otitis externa or a furuncle may call for temporary disqualification. Obstruction of the canal by impacted cerumen or cellular debris may indicate a need for referral to an ENT specialist for examination.

The tympanic membranes should be examined for scars or perforations. Discharge or granulation tissue may be the only observable indication of perforation. Middle ear disease may be revealed by retraction, fluid levels, or discoloration. The normal tympanic membrane is movable and pearly gray in color. Mobility should be demonstrated by watching the drum through the otoscope during a valsalva maneuver.

3. Pathology of the *middle ear* may be demonstrated by changes in the appearance and mobility of the tympanic membrane. The applicant may only complain of stuffiness of the ears and/or loss of hearing. An upper respiratory infection greatly increases the risk of aerotitis media with pain, deafness, tinnitus, and vertigo due to lessened aeration of the middle ear from eustachian tube dysfunction. When the applicant is taking medication for an ENT condition, it is important that the Examiner become fully aware of the underlying pathology, present status, and the length of time the medication has been used. If the condition is not a threat to aviation safety, the treatment consists solely of antibiotics, and the antibiotics have been taken over a sufficient period to rule out the likelihood of adverse side effects, the Examiner may make the certification decision.

The same approach should be taken when considering the significance of prior surgery such as myringotomy, mastoidectomy, or tympanoplasty. Simple perforation without associated symptoms or pathology is not disqualifying. When in doubt, the Examiner should not hesitate to defer issuance and refer the matter to the AMCD. The services of consultant ENT specialists are available to the FAA to help in determining the safety implications of complicated conditions.

4. **Unilateral Deafness.** An applicant with unilateral cogenital or acquired deafness should not be denied medical certification if able to pass any of the tests of hearing acuity.

5. **Bilateral Deafness.** It is possible for a totally deaf person to qualify for a private pilot certificate. When such an applicant initially applies for medical certification, if otherwise qualified, the AMCD may issue a combination medical/student pilot certificate with the limitation "Valid for Student Pilot Purposes Only." This will allow the student to practice with an instructor before undergoing a pilot check ride for the private pilot's license. When the applicant is ready to take the check ride, he/she must contact AMCD or the RFS for authorization to take a medical flight test (MFT). Upon successful completion of the MFT, the applicant will be issued a SODA, and an operational restriction will be placed on his/her pilot's license that restricts the pilot from flying into airspace requiring radio communication.

6. **Hearing Aids.** Under some circumstances, the use of hearing aids may be acceptable. If the applicant is unable to pass any of the above tests without the use of hearing aids, he or she may be tested using hearing aids.

7. The *nose* should be examined for the presence of polyps, blood, or signs of infection, allergy, or substance abuse. The Examiner should determine if there is a

history of epistaxis with exposure to high altitudes and if there is any indication of loss of sense of smell (anosmia). Polyps may cause airway obstruction or sinus blockage. Infection or allergy may be cause for obtaining additional history. Anosmia is at least noteworthy in that the airman should be made fully aware of the significance of the handicap in flying (inability to receive early warning of gas spills, oil leaks, or smoke). Further evaluation may be warranted.

8. Evidence of **sinus** disease must be carefully evaluated by a specialist because of the risk of sudden and severe incapacitation from barotrauma.

9. The **mouth and throat** should be examined to determine the presence of active disease that is progressive or may interfere with voice communications. Gross abnormalities that could interfere with the use of personal equipment such as oxygen equipment should be identified.

10. The **larynx** should be visualized if the applicant's voice is rough or husky. Acute laryngitis is temporarily disqualifying. Chronic laryngitis requires further diagnostic workup. Any applicant seeking certification for the first time with a functioning tracheostomy, following laryngectomy, or who uses an artificial voice-producing device should be denied or deferred and carefully assessed.

III. Aerospace Medical Disposition

The following is a table that lists the most common conditions of aeromedical significance, and course of action that should be taken by the examiner as defined by the protocol and disposition in the table. Medical certificates must not be issued to an applicant with medical conditions that require deferral, or for any condition not listed in the table that may result in sudden or subtle incapacitation without consulting the AMCD or the RFS. Medical documentation must be submitted for any condition in order to support an issuance of an airman medical certificate.

ITEM 25. Head, Face, Neck, and Scalp

DISEASE/CONDITION	CLASS	EVALUATION DATA	DISPOSITION
Head, Face, Neck, and Scalp			
Active fistula of neck, either congenital or acquired, including tracheostomy	All	Submit all pertinent medical information and current status report	Requires FAA Decision
Loss of bony substance involving the two tables of the cranial vault	All	Submit all pertinent medical information and current status report	Requires FAA Decision
Deformities of the face or head that would interfere with the proper fitting and wearing of an oxygen mask	1st & 2nd	Submit all pertinent medical information and current status report	Requires FAA Decision
	3rd	Submit all pertinent medical information	If deformity does not interfere with administration of supplemental O² - Issue

ITEM 26. Nose

DISEASE/CONDITION	CLASS	EVALUATION DATA	DISPOSITION
Nose			
Evidence of severe allergic rhinitis[1]	All	Submit all pertinent medical information and current status report	Requires FAA Decision

---

[1] Hay fever controlled solely by desensitization without requiring antihistamines or other medications is not disqualifying. Applicants with seasonal allergies requiring antihistamines may be certified by the Examiner with the stipulation that they not exercise privileges of airman certification within 24 hours of experiencing symptoms requiring treatment or within 24 hours after taking an antihistamine. The Examiner should document this in **Item 60**. However, non-sedating antihistamines loratadine or fexofenadine may be used while flying, after adequate individual experience has determined that the medication is well tolerated without significant side effects.

DISEASE/CONDITION	CLASS	EVALUATION DATA	DISPOSITION
Nose			
Obstruction of sinus ostia, including polyps, that would be likely to result in complete obstruction	All	Submit all pertinent medical information and current status report	Requires FAA Decision

ITEM 27. Sinuses

DISEASE/CONDITION	CLASS	EVALUATION DATA	DISPOSITION
Sinuses - Acute or Chronic			
Sinusitis, intermittent use of topical or non-sedating medication	All	Document medication, dose and absence of side effects	Responds to treatment without any side effects - Issue
Severe-requiring continuous use of medication or effected by barometric changes	All	Submit all pertinent medical information and current status report	Requires FAA Decision
Sinus Tumor			
Benign - Cysts/Polyps	All	If no physiologic effects, submit documentation	Asymptomatic, no observable growth over a 12-month period, no potential for sinus block - Issue
Malignant	All	Submit all pertinent medical information and current status report	Requires FAA Decision

ITEM 28. Mouth and Throat

DISEASE/CONDITION	CLASS	EVALUATION DATA	DISPOSITION
Mouth and Throat			
Any malformation or condition, including stuttering, that would impair voice communication	All	Submit all pertinent medical information and current status report	Requires FAA Decision
Palate: Extensive adhesion of the soft palate to the pharynx	All	Submit all pertinent medical information and current status report	Requires FAA Decision

ITEM 29. Ears, General

DISEASE/CONDITION	CLASS	EVALUATION DATA	DISPOSITION
Inner Ear			
Acoustic Neuroma	All	Submit all pertinent medical information and current status report	Requires FAA Decision
Acute or chronic disease without disturbance of equilibrium and successful miringotomy, if applicable	All	Submit all pertinent medical information	If no physiologic effects - Issue
Acute or chronic disease that may disturb equilibrium	All	Submit all pertinent medical information and current status report	Requires FAA Decision
Motion Sickness	All	Submit all pertinent medical information and current status report	If occurred during flight training and resolved - Issue If condition requires medication - Requires FAA Decision

DISEASE/CONDITION	CLASS	EVALUATION DATA	DISPOSITION
Mastoids			
Mastoid fistula	All	Submit all pertinent medical information and current status report	Requires FAA Decision
Mastoiditis, acute or chronic	All	Submit all pertinent medical information and current status report	Requires FAA Decision
Middle Ear			
Impaired Aeration	All	Submit all pertinent medical information and current status report	Requires FAA Decision
Otitis Media	All	Submit all pertinent medical information and current status report	If acute and resolved – Issue If active or chronic - Requires FAA Decision
Outer Ear			
Impacted Cerumen	All	Submit all pertinent medical information and current status report	If asymptomatic and hearing is unaffected - Issue Otherwise - Requires FAA Decision
Otitis Externa that may progress to impaired hearing or become incapacitating	All	Submit all pertinent medical information and current status report	Requires FAA Decision

ITEM 30. Ear Drums

DISEASE/CONDITION	CLASS	EVALUATION DATA	DISPOSITION
Ear Drums			
Perforation that has associated pathology	All	Establish etiology, treatment, and submit all pertinent medical information	Requires FAA Decision
Perforation which has resolved without any other clinical symptoms	All	Submit all pertinent medical information	If no physiologic effects - Issue

Otologic Surgery. A history of otologic surgery is not necessarily disqualifying for medical certification. The FAA evaluates each case on an individual basis following review of the otologist's report of surgery. The type of prosthesis used, the person's adaptability and progress following surgery, and the extent of hearing acuity attained are all major factors to be considered. Examiners should defer issuance to an applicant presenting a history of otologic surgery for the first time, sending the completed report of medical examination, with all available supplementary information, to the AMCD. Some conditions may have several possible causes or exhibit multiple symptomatology. Episodic disorders of dizziness or disequilibrium require careful evaluation and consideration by the FAA. Transient processes, such as those associated with acute labyrinthitis or benign positional vertigo may not disqualify an applicant when fully recovered. (Also see **Item 46., Neurologic** for a discussion of syncope and vertigo).

ITEMS 31-34. Eye

CHECK EACH ITEM IN APPROPRIATE COLUMN	Normal	Abnormal
31. Eyes, general (vision under Items 50 to 54)		
32. Ophthalmoscopic		
33. Pupils (Equity and reaction)		
34. Ocular motility (Associated parallel movement nystagmus)		

I. Code of Federal Regulations

All Classes: 14 CFR 67.103(e), 67.203(e), and 67.303(d)

(e) No acute or chronic pathological condition of either the eye or adnexa that interferes with the proper function of the eye, that may reasonably be expected to progress to that degree, or that may reasonably be expected to be aggravated by flying.

II. Examination Techniques

For guidance regarding the conduct of visual acuity, field of vision, heterophoria, and color vision tests, please see **Items 50-54**.

The examination of the eyes should be directed toward the discovery of diseases or defects that may cause a failure in visual function while flying or discomfort sufficient to interfere with safely performing airman duties.

The Examiner should personally explore the applicant's history by asking questions concerning any changes in vision, unusual visual experiences (halos, scintillations, etc.), sensitivity to light, injuries, surgery, or current use of medication. Does the applicant report inordinate difficulties with eye fatigue or strain? Is there a history of serious eye disease such as glaucoma or other disease commonly associated with secondary eye changes, such as diabetes? (See **Item 53., Field of Vision** and **Item 54., Heterophoria**)

1. It is recommended that the Examiner consider the following signs during the course of the eye examination:

   1. *Color* — redness or suffusion of allergy, drug use, glaucoma, infection, trauma, jaundice, ciliary flush of Iritis, and the green or brown Kayser-Fleischer Ring of Wilson's disease.

   2. *Swelling* — abscess, allergy, cyst, exophthalmos, myxedema, or tumor.

   3. *Other* — clarity, discharge, dryness, ptosis, protosis, spasm (tic), tropion, or ulcer.

2. Ophthalmoscopic examination. It is suggested that a routine be established for ophthalmoscopic examinations to aid in the conduct of a comprehensive eye assessment. Routine use of a mydriatic is not recommended.

   a. *Cornea* — observe for abrasions, calcium deposits, contact lenses, dystrophy, keratoconus, pterygium, scars, or ulceration. Contact lenses should be removed several hours before examination of the eye. (See **Item 50, Distant Vision**)

   b. *Pupils and Iris* — check for the presence of synechiae and uveitis. Size, shape, and reaction to light should be evaluated during the ophthalmoscopic examination. Observe for coloboma, reaction to light, or disparity in size.

   c. *Aqueous* — hyphema or iridocyclitis.

d. *Lens* — observe for aphakia, discoloration, dislocation, cataract, or an implanted lens.

e. *Vitreous* — note discoloration, hyaloid artery, floaters, or strands.

f. *Optic nerve* — observe for atrophy, hemorrhage, cupping, or papilledema.

g. *Retina and choroid* — examine for evidence of coloboma, choroiditis, detachment of the retina, diabetic retinopathy, retinitis, retinitis pigmentosa, retinal tumor, macular or other degeneration, toxoplasmosis, etc.

3. Ocular Motility. Motility may be assessed by having the applicant follow a point light source with both eyes, the Examiner moving the light into right and left upper and lower quadrants while observing the individual and the conjugate motions of each eye. The Examiner then brings the light to center front and advances it toward the nose observing for convergence. End point nystagmus is a physiologic nystagmus and is not considered to be significant. It need not be reported. (For further consideration of nystagmus, see **Item 50., Distant Vision**.)

4. Monocular Vision. An applicant will be considered monocular when there is only one eye or when the best corrected distant visual acuity in the poorer eye is no better than 20/200. An individual with one eye, or effective visual acuity equivalent to monocular, may be considered for medical certification, any class, through the special issuance section of part 67 (14 CFR 67.401).

In amblyopia ex anopsia, the visual acuity loss is simply recorded in Item 50 of FAA Form 8500-8, and visual standards are applied as usual. If the standards are not met, a Report of Eye Evaluation, FAA Form 8500-7, should be submitted for consideration.

Although it has been repeatedly demonstrated that binocular vision is not a prerequisite for flying, some aspects of depth perception, either by stereopsis or by monocular cues, are necessary. It takes time for the monocular airman to develop the techniques to interpret the monocular cues that substitute for stereopsis; such as, the interposition of objects, convergence, geometrical perspective, distribution of light and shade, size of known objects, aerial perspective, and motion parallax.

In addition, it takes time for the monocular airman to compensate for his or her decrease in effective visual field. A monocular airman's effective visual field is reduced by as much as 30% by monocularity. This is especially important because of speed smear; i.e., the effect of speed diminishes the effective visual field such that normal visual field is decreased from 180 degrees to as narrow as 42 degrees or less as speed increases. A monocular airman's reduced effective visual field would be reduced even further than 42 degrees by speed smear.

For the above reasons, a waiting period of 6 months is recommended to permit an adequate adjustment period for learning techniques to interpret monocular cues and accommodation to the reduction in the effective visual field.

Applicants who have had monovision secondary to refractive surgery may be certificated, providing they have corrective vision available that would provide binocular vision in accordance with the vision standards, while exercising the privileges of the certificate. The certificate issued must have the appropriate vision limitations statement.

5. Contact Lenses. The use of contact lens(es) for monovision correction is not allowed:

- The use of a contact lens in one eye for near vision and in the other eye for distant vision is not acceptable (for example: pilots with myopia plus presbyopia).

- The use of a contact lens in one eye for near vision and the use of no contact lens in the other eye is not acceptable (for example: pilots with presbyopia but no myopia).

Additionally, designer contact lenses that introduce color (tinted lenses), restrict the field of vision, or significantly diminish transmitted light are not allowed.

Please note: the use of binocular contact lenses for distance-correction-only is acceptable. In this instance, no special evaluation or SODA is routinely required for a distance-vision-only contact lens wearer who meets the standard and has no complications. Binocular bifocal or binocular multifocal contact lenses are acceptable under the Protocol for Binocular Multifocal and Accommodating Devices.

6. Intraocular Devices. Binocular airman using multifocal or accommodating ophthalmic devices may be issued an airman medical certificate in accordance with the Protocol for Binocular Multifocal and Accommodating Devices.

7. Orthokeratology (Ortho-K) is the use of rigid gas-permeable contact lenses, normally worn only during sleep, to improve vision through reshaping of the cornea. It is used as an alternative to eyeglasses, refractive surgery, or for those who prefer not to wear contact lenses while awake. The correction is not permanent and visual acuity can regress while not wearing the Ortho-K lenses. There is no reasonable or reliable way to determine standards for the entire period the lenses are removed. Therefore, to be found qualified, applicants who use Ortho-K lenses **must meet the applicable vision standard while wearing the Ortho-K lenses AND must wear the Ortho-K lenses while piloting aircraft.** The limitation "must use Ortho-K lenses while performing pilot duties" must be placed on the medical certificate.

8. Glaucoma. The Examiner should deny or defer issuance of a medical certificate to an applicant if there is a loss of visual fields, a significant change in visual acuity, a diagnosis of or treatment for glaucoma, or newly diagnosed intraocular hypertension.

The FAA may grant an Authorization under the special issuance section of Part 67 (14 CFR 67.401) on an individual basis. The Examiner can facilitate FAA review by obtaining a report of Ophthalmological Evaluation for Glaucoma (FAA Form 8500-14) from a treating or evaluating eye specialist (optometrist or ophthmologist), also see AME assisted protocol. Because secondary glaucoma is caused by known pathology such as; uveitis or trauma, eligibility must largely depend upon that pathology. Secondary glaucoma is often unilateral, and if the cause or disease process is no longer active and the other eye remains normal certification is likely.

Applicants with primary or secondary narrow angle glaucoma are usually denied because of the risk of an attack of angle closure, because of incapacitating symptoms of severe pain, nausea, transitory loss of accommodative power, blurred vision, halos, epiphora, or iridoparesis. Central venous occlusion can occur with catastrophic loss of vision. However, when surgery such as iridectomy or iridencleisis has been performed satisfactorily more than 3 months before the application, the likelihood of difficulties is considerably more remote, and applicants in that situation may be favorably considered by the FAA.

An applicant with unilateral or bilateral open angle glaucoma may be certified by the FAA (with follow-up required) when a current ophthalmological report substantiates that pressures are under adequate control, there is little or no visual field loss or other complications, and the person tolerates small to moderate doses of allowable medications. Individuals who have had filter surgery for their glaucoma, or combined glaucoma/cataract surgery, can be considered when stable and without complications. A few applicants have been certified following their demonstration of adequate control with oral medication. Neither miotics nor mydriatics are necessarily medically disqualifying.

However, miotics such as pilocarpine cause pupillary constriction and could conceivably interfere with night vision. Although the FAA no longer routinely prohibits pilots who use such medications from flying at night, it may be worthwhile for the Examiner to discuss this aspect of the use of miotics with applicants. If considerable disturbance in night vision is documented, the FAA may limit the medical certificate: NOT VALID FOR NIGHT FLYING

9. Sunglasses. Sunglasses are not acceptable as the only means of correction to meet visual standards, but may be used for backup purposes if they provide the necessary correction. Airmen should be encouraged to use sunglasses in bright daylight but must be cautioned that, under conditions of low illumination, they may compromise vision. Mention should be made that sunglasses do not protect

the eyes from the effects of ultra violet radiation without special glass or coatings and that photosensitive lenses are unsuitable for aviation purposes because they respond to changes in light intensity too slowly. The so-called "blue blockers" may not be suitable since they block the blue light used in many current panel displays. Polarized sunglasses are unacceptable if the windscreen is also polarized.

10. Refractive Procedures. The FAA accepts the following Food and Drug Administration approved refractive procedures for visual acuity correction:

- Radial Keratotomy (RK)
- Epikeratophakia
- Laser-Assisted In Situ Keratomileusis (LASIK), including Wavefront-guided LASIK
- Photorefractive Keratectomy (PRK)
- Conductive Keratoplasty (CK)

Please be advised that these procedures have potential adverse effects that could be incompatible with flying duties, including: corneal scarring or opacities; worsening or variability of vision; and night-glare.

The FAA expects that airmen will not resume airman duties until their treating health care professional determines that their post-operative vision has stabilized, there are no significant adverse effects or complications (such as halos, rings, haze, impaired night vision and glare), the appropriate vision standards are met, and reviewed by an Examiner or AMCD. When this determination is made, the airman should have the treating health care professional document this in the health care record, a copy of which should be forwarded to the AMCD before resumption of airman duties. If the health care professional's determination is favorable, the applicant may resume airman duties, after consultation and review by an Examiner, unless informed otherwise by the FAA.

An applicant treated with a refractive procedure may be issued a medical certificate by the Examiner if the applicant meets the visual acuity standards and the Report of Eye Evaluation (FAA Form 8500-7) indicates that healing is complete; visual acuity remains stable; and the applicant does not suffer sequela such as; glare intolerance, halos, rings, impaired night vision, or any other complications. There should be no other pathology of the affected eye(s).

If the procedure was done 2 years ago or longer, the FAA may accept the Examiner's eye evaluation and an airman statement regarding the absence of adverse sequela.

If the procedure was performed within the last 2 years, the airman must provide a report to the AMCD from the treating health care professional to document the date of procedure, any adverse effects or complications, and when the airman returned to flying duties. If the report is favorable and the airman meets the appropriate vision standards, the applicant may resume airman duties, unless informed otherwise by the FAA.

A. Conductive Keratoplasty (CK): CK is used for correction of farsightedness. As this procedure is not considered permanent and there is expected regression of visual acuity in time, the FAA may grant an Authorization for special issuance of a medical certificate under 14 CFR 67.401 to an applicant who has had CK.

The FAA evaluates CK procedures on an individual basis following a waiting period of 6 months. The waiting period is required to permit adequate adjustment period for fluctuating visual acuity. The Examiner can facilitate FAA review by obtaining all pre- and post-operative medical records, a Report of Eye Evaluation (FAA Form 8500-7) from a treating or evaluating eye specialist with comment regarding any adverse effects or complications related to the procedure.

III. Aerospace Medical Disposition

Applicants with many visual conditions may be found qualified for FAA certification following the receipt and review of specialty evaluations and pertinent medical records. Examples include retinal detachment with surgical correction, open angle glaucoma under adequate control with medication, and narrow angle glaucoma following surgical correction.

The Examiner may not issue a certificate under such circumstances for the initial application, except in the case of applicants following cataract surgery. The Examiner may issue a certificate after cataract surgery for applicants who have undergone cataract surgery with or without lens(es) implant. If pertinent medical records and a current ophthalmologic evaluation (using FAA Form 8500-7 or FAA Form 8500-14) indicate that the applicant meets the standards, the FAA may delegate authority to the Examiner to issue subsequent certificates.

The following is a table that lists the most common conditions of aeromedical significance, and course of action that should be taken by the examiner as defined by the protocol and disposition in the table. Medical certificates must not be issued to an applicant with medical conditions that require deferral, or for any condition not listed in the table that may result in sudden or subtle incapacitation without consulting the AMCD or the RFS. Medical documentation must be submitted for any condition in order to support an issuance of an airman medical certificate.

ITEM 31. Eyes, General

DISEASE/CONDITION	CLASS	EVALUTION DATA	DISPOSITION
Eyes, General			
Amblyopia[1] Initial certification	All	Provide completed FAA Form 8500-7 Note: applicant should be at best corrected visual acuity before evaluation	If applicant does not correct to standards, add the following limitation to the medical certificate: "Valid for Student Pilot Purposes Only" and request a medical flight test
Congenital or acquired conditions (whether acute or chronic) of either eye or adnexa, that may interfere with visual functions, may progress to that degree, or may be aggravated by flying (tumors and ptosis obscuring the pupil, acute inflammatory disease of the eyes and lids, cataracts, or keratoconus.)	All	Provide completed FAA Form 8500-7 Submit all pertinent medical information and current status report For keratoconus, include if available results of imaging studies such as kertatometry, videokeratography, etc., with clinical correlation Note: applicant should be at best corrected visual acuity before evaluation	Requires FAA Decision
Any ophthalmic pathology reflecting a serious systemic disease (e.g., diabetic and hypertensive retinopathy)	All	Submit all pertinent medical information and current status report. (If applicable, see Diabetes and Hypertensive Protocols)	Requires FAA Decision
Diplopia	All	If applicant provides written evidence that the FAA has previously considered and determined that this condition is not adverse to flight safety. A MFT may be	Contact RFS for approval to Issue Otherwise - Requires FAA Decision

[1] In amblyopia ex anopsia, the visual acuity of one eye is decreased without presence of organic eye disease, usually because of strabismus or anisometropia in childhood.

DISEASE/CONDITION	CLASS	EVALUATION DATA	DISPOSITION
		requested.	
Pterygium	All	Document findings in Item 60	If less than 50% of the cornea and not affecting central vision - Issue Otherwise - Requires FAA Decision

Eyes - Procedures

DISEASE/CONDITION	CLASS	EVALUATION DATA	DISPOSITION
Aphakia/Lens Implants	All	Submit all pertinent medical information and current status report (See additional disease dependent requirements)	If visual acuity meets standards - Issue Otherwise - Requires FAA Decision
Conductive Keratoplasty - Farsightedness	All	See Protocol for Conductive Keratoplasty	See Protocol for Conductive Keratoplasty
Intraocular Devices	All	See Protocol for Binocular Multifocal and Accommodating Devices	See Protocol for Binocular Multifocal and Accommodating Devices
Refractive Procedures other than CK	All	Provide completed FAA Form 8500-7, type and date of procedure, statement as to any adverse effects or complications (halo, glare, haze, rings, etc.)	If visual acuity meets standards, is stable, and no complications exist - Issue Otherwise - Requires FAA Decision

ITEM 32. Ophthalmoscopic

DISEASE/CONDITION	CLASS	EVALUATION DATA	DISPOSITION
Ophthalmoscopic			
Chorioretinitis; Coloboma; Corneal Ulcer or Dystrophy; Optic Atrophy or Neuritis; Retinal Degeneration or Detachment; Retinitis Pigmentosa; Papilledema; or Uveitis	All	Submit all pertinent medical information and current status report	Requires FAA Decision
Glaucoma (treated or untreated)	All	Submit all pertinent medical information and current status report including Form 8500-14	**Initial Special Issuance** - Requires FAA Decision **Followup Special Issuance's** - See AASI Protocol
Macular Degeneration; Macular Detachment	All	Submit all pertinent medical information and current status report	Requires FAA Decision
Tumors	All	Submit all pertinent medical information and current status report	Requires FAA Decision
Vascular Occlusion; Retinopathy	All	Submit all pertinent medical information and current status report	Requires FAA Decision

ITEM 33. Pupils

DISEASE/CONDITION	CLASS	EVALUATION DATA	DISPOSITION
Pupils			
Disparity in size or reaction to light (afferent pupillary defect) requires clarification and/or	All	Submit all pertinent medical information and current status report	Requires FAA Decision

DISEASE/CONDITION	CLASS	EVALUATION DATA	DISPOSITION
further evaluation			
Pupils			
Nonreaction to light in either eye acute or chronic	All	Submit all pertinent medical information and current status report	Requires FAA Decision
Nystagmus[1]	All	Submit all pertinent medical information and current status report	Requires FAA Decision
Synechiae, anterior or posterior	All	Submit all pertinent medical information and current status report	Requires FAA Decision

ITEM 34. Ocular Motility

DISEASE/CONDITION	CLASS	EVALUATION DATA	DISPOSITION
Ocular Motility			
Absence of conjugate alignment in any quadrant	All	Submit all pertinent medical information and current status report	Requires FAA Decision
Inability to converge on a near object	All	Submit all pertinent medical information and current status report	Requires FAA Decision
Paralysis with loss of ocular motion in any direction	All	Submit all pertinent medical information and current status report	Requires FAA Decision

---

[1] Nystagmus of recent onset is cause to deny or defer certificate issuance. Any recent neurological or other evaluations available to the Examiner should be submitted to the AMCD. If nystagmus has been present for a number of years and has not recently worsened, it is usually necessary to consider only the impact that the nystagmus has upon visual acuity. The Examiner should be aware of how nystagmus may be aggravated by the forces of acceleration commonly encountered in aviation and by poor illumination.

ITEM 35. Lungs and Chest

CHECK EACH ITEM IN APPROPRIATE COLUMN	Normal	Abnormal
35. Lungs and chest (Not including breasts examination)		

I. Code of Federal Regulations

All Classes: 14 CFR 67.113(b)(c), 67.213(b)(c), and 67.313(b)(c)

(b) No other organic, functional, or structural disease, defect, or limitation that the Federal Air Surgeon, based on the case history and appropriate, qualified medical judgment relating to the condition involved, finds -

(1) Makes the person unable to safely perform the duties or exercise the privileges of the airman certificate applied for or held; or

(2) May reasonably be expected, for the maximum duration of the airman medical certificate applied for or held, to make the person unable to perform those duties or exercise those privileges;

(c) No medication or other treatment that the Federal Air Surgeon, based on the case history and appropriate, qualified medical judgment relating to the medication or other treatment involved, finds -

(1) Makes the person unable to safely perform the duties or exercise the privileges of the airman certificate applied for or held; or

(2) May reasonably be expected, for the maximum duration of the airman medical certificate applied for or held, to make the person unable to perform those duties or exercise those privileges.

II. Examination Techniques

Breast examination: The breast examination is performed only at the applicant's option or if indicated by specific history or physical findings. If a breast examination is performed, the results are to be recorded in Item 60 of FAA Form 8500-8. The applicant should be advised of any abnormality that is detected, then deferred for further evaluation.

III. Aerospace Medical Dispositions

The following is a table that lists the most common conditions of aeromedical significance, and course of action that should be taken by the examiner as defined by the protocol and disposition in the table. Medical certificates must not be issued to an applicant with medical conditions that require deferral, or for any condition not listed in the table that may result in sudden or subtle incapacitation without consulting the AMCD or the RFS. Medical documentation must be submitted for any condition in order to support an issuance of an airman medical certificate.

DISEASE/CONDITION	CLASS	EVALUATION DATA	DISPOSITION
Allergies			
Allergies, severe	All	Submit all pertinent medical information and current status report, include duration of symptoms, name and dosage of drugs and side effects	Requires FAA Decision
Hay fever controlled solely by desensitization without antihistamines or other medications[1] [2] [3]	All	Submit all pertinent medical information and current status report, include duration of symptoms, name and dosage of drugs and side effects	If responds to treatment and without side effects - Issue Otherwise - Requires FAA Decision

[1] Applicants with seasonal allergies requiring antihistamines may be certified by the Examiner with the stipulation that they not exercise privileges of airman certification within 24 hours of experiencing symptoms requiring treatment or within 24 hours after taking an antihistamine. The Examiner should document this in Item 60.

[2] Individuals who have hay fever that requires only occasional seasonal therapy may be certified by the Examiner with the stipulation that they not fly during the time when symptoms occur and treatment is required.

[3] Nonsedating antihistamines including loratadine, or fexofenadine may be used while flying, after adequate individual experience has determined that the medication is well tolerated without significant side effects.

DISEASE/CONDITION	CLASS	EVALUATION DATA	DISPOSITION
Asthma			
Frequent severe asthmatic symptoms	All	Submit all pertinent medical information and current status report, include PFT's, duration of symptoms, name and dosage of drugs and side effects	**Initial Special Issuance** - Requires FAA Decision **Followup Special Issuance's** - See AASI Protocol
Mild or seasonal asthmatic symptoms[4]	All	Submit all pertinent medical information and current status report, include duration of symptoms, name and dosage of drugs, and side effects	If symptoms are infrequent, mild, have not required hospitalization or steroid medication, and no symptoms in flight – Issue

---

[4] If the applicant otherwise meets the medical standards and currently requires no treatment, the Examiner may Issue. However, a history of frequent severe attacks is disqualifying. Certificate issuance may be possible in other cases. If additional information is obtained, it must be submitted to the FAA.

DISEASE/CONDITION	CLASS	EVALUATION DATA	DISPOSITION
Chronic Obstructive Pulmonary Disease (COPD)			
Chronic bronchitis, emphysema, or COPD[5]	All	Submit all pertinent medical information and current status report. Include an FVC/FEV1	**Initial Special Issuance** - Requires FAA Decision **Followup Special Issuance's** - See AASI Protocol
Disease of the Lungs, Pleura, or Mediastinum			
Abscesses Active Mycotic disease Active Tuberculosis	All	Submit all pertinent medical information and current status report	Requires FAA Decision
Fistula, Bronchopleural, to include Thoracostomy	All	Submit all pertinent medical information and current status report	Requires FAA Decision
Lobectomy	All	Submit all pertinent medical information and current status report	Requires FAA Decision
Pulmonary Embolism	All	See Thromboembolic Disease Protocol	See Thromboembolic Disease Protocol
Pulmonary Fibrosis	All	Submit all pertinent medical information, current status report, PFT's with diffusion capacity	If >75% predicted and no impairment - Issue Otherwise - Requires FAA Decision

---

[5] Certification may be granted, by the FAA, when the condition is mild without significant impairment of pulmonary functions. If the applicant has frequent exacerbations or any degree of exertional dyspnea, certification should be deferred.

DISEASE/CONDITION	CLASS	EVALUATION DATA	DISPOSITION
Pleura and Pleural Cavity			
Acute fibrinous pleurisy; Empyema; Pleurisy with effusion; or Pneumonectomy	All	Submit all pertinent medical information and current status report, and PFT's	Requires FAA Decision
Malignant tumors or cysts of the lung, pleura or mediastinum	All	Submit all pertinent medical information and current status report	Requires FAA Decision
Other diseases or defects of the lungs or chest wall that require use of medication or that could adversely affect flying or endanger the applicant's well-being if permitted to fly	All	Submit all pertinent medical information and current status report	Requires FAA Decision
Pneumothorax - Traumatic	All	Submit all pertinent medical information and current status report	If 3 months after resolution - Issue
Sarcoid, if more than minimal involvement or if symptomatic	All	Submit all pertinent medical information and current status report	Requires FAA Decision
Spontaneous pneumothorax [6]	All	Submit all pertinent medical information and current status report	Requires FAA Decision

[6] A history of a single episode of spontaneous pneumothorax is considered disqualifying for airman medical certification until there is x-ray evidence of resolution and until it can be determined that no condition that would be likely to cause recurrence is present (i.e., residual blebs). On the other hand, an individual who has sustained a repeat pneumothorax normally is not eligible for certification until surgical interventions are carried out to correct the underlying problem. A person who has such a history is usually able to resume airmen duties 3 months after the surgery. No special limitations on flying at altitude are applied.

DISEASE/CONDITION	CLASS	EVALUATION DATA	DISPOSITION
Pulmonary			
Bronchiectasis	All	Submit all pertinent medical information and current status report	If moderate to severe - Requires FAA Decision
Sleep Apnea			
Obstructive Sleep Apnea	All	Submit all pertinent medical information and current status report. Include sleep study with a polysomnogram, use of medications and titration study results	**Initial Special Issuance** - Requires FAA Decision **Followup Special Issuance's** - See AASI Protocol
Periodic Limb Movement, etc.	All	Submit all pertinent medical information and current status report. Include sleep study with a polysomnogram, use of medications and titration study results, along with a statement regarding Restless Leg Syndrome	Requires FAA Decision

ITEM 36. Heart

CHECK EACH ITEM IN APPROPRIATE COLUMN	Normal	Abnormal
36. Heart (Precordial activity, rhythm, sounds, and murmurs)		

I. Code of Federal Regulations:

First-Class: 14 CFR 67.111(a)(b)(c)

Cardiovascular standards for first-class airman medical certificate are:

(a) No established medical history or clinical diagnosis of any of the following:

(1) Myocardial infarction

(2) Angina pectoris

(3) Coronary heart disease that has required treatment or, if untreated, that has been symptomatic or clinically significant

(4) Cardiac valve replacement

(5) Permanent cardiac pacemaker implantation; or

(6) Heart replacement

(b) A person applying for first-class airman medical certification must demonstrate an absence of myocardial infarction and other clinically significant abnormality on electrocardiographic examination:

(1) At the first application after reaching the 35th birthday; and

(2) On an annual basis after reaching the 40th birthday

(c) An electrocardiogram will satisfy a requirement of paragraph (b) of this section if it is dated no earlier than 60 days before the date of the application it is to accompany and was performed and transmitted according to acceptable standards and techniques.

Second- and Third-Class: 14 CFR 67.211(a)(b)(c)(d)(e)(f) and 67.311(a)(b)(c)(d)(e)(f)

Cardiovascular standards for a second- and third-class airman medical certificate are no established medical history or clinical diagnosis of any of the following:

(a) Myocardial infarction

(b) Angina pectoris

(c) Coronary heart disease that has required treatment or, if untreated, that has been symptomatic or clinically significant

(d) Cardiac valve replacement

(e) Permanent cardiac pacemaker implantation; or

(f) Heart replacement

II. Examination Techniques

A. General Physical Examination.

1. A brief description of any comment-worthy personal characteristics as well as height, weight, representative blood pressure readings in both arms, funduscopic examination, condition of peripheral arteries, carotid artery auscultation, heart size, heart rate, heart rhythm, description of murmurs (location, intensity, timing, and opinion as to significance), and other findings of consequence must be provided.

2. The Examiner should keep in mind some of the special cardiopulmonary demands of flight, such as changes in heart rates at takeoff and landing. High G-forces of aerobatics or agricultural flying may stress both systems considerably. Degenerative changes are often insidious and may produce subtle performance decrements that may require special investigative techniques.

   a. Inspection. Observe and report any thoracic deformity (e.g., pectus excavatum), signs of surgery or other trauma, and clues to ventricular hypertrophy. Check the hematopoietic and vascular system by observing for pallor, edema, varicosities, stasis ulcers, and venous distention. Check the nail beds for capillary pulsation and color.

   b. Palpation. Check for thrills and the vascular system for arteriosclerotic changes, shunts, or AV anastomoses. The pulses should be examined to determine their character, to note if they are diminished or absent, and to observe for synchronicity. The medical standards do not specify pulse rates that, per se, are disqualifying for medical certification. These tests are used, however, to determine the status and responsiveness of the cardiovascular system. Abnormal pulse rates may be reason to conduct additional cardiovascular system evaluations.

    i. Bradycardia of less than 50 beats per minute, any episode of tachycardia during the course of the examination, and any other irregularities of pulse other than an occasional ectopic beat or sinus arrhythmia must be noted and reported. If there is bradycardia, tachycardia, or arrhythmia further evaluation may be warranted and deferral may be indicated.

    ii. A cardiac evaluation may be needed to determine the applicant's qualifications. Temporary stresses or fever may, at times, result in abnormal results from these tests. If the Examiner believes this to be the case, the applicant should be given a few days to recover and then be retested. If this is not possible, the Examiner should defer issuance, pending further evaluation.

c. Percussion. Determine heart size, diaphragmatic elevation/excursion, abnormal densities in the pulmonary fields, and mediastinal shift.

d. Auscultation. Check for resonance, asthmatic wheezing, ronchi, rales, cavernous breathing of emphysema, pulmonary or pericardial friction rubs, quality of the heart sounds, murmurs, heart rate, and rhythm. If a murmur is discovered during the course of conducting a routine FAA examination, report its character, loudness, timing, transmission, and change with respiration. It should be noted whether it is functional or organic and if a special examination is needed. If the latter is indicated, the Examiner should defer issuance of the medical certificate and transmit the completed FAA Form 8500-8 to the FAA for further consideration. Examiner must defer to the AMCD or Region if the treating physician or Examiner reports the murmur is moderate to severe (Grade III or IV). Listen to the neck for bruits.

It is recommended that the Examiner conduct the auscultation of the heart with the applicant both in a sitting and in a recumbent position.

Aside from murmur, irregular rhythm, and enlargement, the Examiner should be careful to observe for specific signs that are pathognomonic for specific disease entities or for serious generalized heart disease. Examples of such evidence are: (1) the opening snap at the apex or fourth left intercostal space signifying mitral stenosis; (2) gallop rhythm indicating serious impairment of cardiac function; and (3) the middiastolic rumble of mitral stenosis.

B. When General Examinations Reveal Heart Problems.

These specifications have been developed by the FAA to determine an applicant's eligibility for airman medical certification. Standardization of examination methods and reporting is essential to provide sufficient basis for making determinations and the prompt processing of applications.

1. This cardiovascular evaluation, therefore, must be reported in sufficient detail to permit a clear and objective evaluation of the cardiovascular disorder(s) with emphasis on the degree of functional recovery and prognosis. It should be forwarded to the FAA immediately upon completion. Inadequate evaluation, reporting, or failure to promptly submit the report to the FAA may delay the certification decision.

    a. Medical History. Particular reference should be given to cardiovascular abnormalities-cerebral, visceral, and/or peripheral. A statement must be included as to whether medications are currently or have been recently used, and if so, the type, purpose, dosage, duration of use, and other pertinent details must be provided. A specific history of any anticoagulant drug therapy is required. In addition, any history of hypertension must be fully developed to also include all medications used, dosages, and comments on side effects.

    b. Family, Personal, and Social History. A statement of the ages and health status of parents and siblings is required; if deceased, cause and age at death should be included. Also, any indication of whether any near blood relative has had a "heart attack," hypertension, diabetes, or known disorder of lipid metabolism must be provided. Smoking, drinking, and recreational habits of the applicant are pertinent as well as whether a program of physical fitness is being maintained. Comments on the level of physical activities, functional limitations, occupational, and avocational pursuits are essential.

    c. Records of Previous Medical Care. If not previously furnished to the FAA, a copy of pertinent hospital records as well as out-patient treatment records with clinical data, x-ray, laboratory observations, and originals or copies of all electrocardiographic (ECG) tracings should be provided. Detailed reports of surgical procedures as well as cerebral and coronary arteriography and other major diagnostic studies are of prime importance.

    d. Surgery. The presence of an aneurysm or obstruction of a major vessel of the body is disqualifying for medical certification of any class. Following successful surgical intervention and correction, the applicant may ask for FAA consideration. The FAA recommends that the applicant recover for at least 3 months for ATCS's and 6 months for airmen.

A history of coronary artery bypass surgery is disqualifying for certification. Such surgery does not negate a past history of coronary heart disease. The presence of permanent cardiac pacemakers and artificial heart valves is also disqualifying for certification.

The FAA will consider an Authorization for a Special Issuance of a Medical Certificate (Authorization) for most cardiac conditions. Applicants seeking further FAA consideration should be prepared to submit all past records and a report of a complete current cardiovascular evaluation in accordance with FAA specifications.

C. Medication.

- Medications acceptable to the FAA for treatment of hypertension in airmen include all Food and Drug Administration (FDA) approved diuretics, alpha-adrenergic blocking agents, beta-adrenergic blocking agents, calcium channel blocking agents, angiotension converting enzyme (ACE inhibitors) agents, and direct vasodilators.
- The following are **NOT ACCEPTABLE** to the FAA:
  - Centrally acting agents (such as reserpine, guanethidine, guanadrel, guanabenz, and methyldopa).
  - A combination of beta-adrenergic blocking agents used with insulin, meglitinides, or sulfonylureas.
  - The use of flecainide when there is evidence of left ventricular dysfunction or recent myocardial infarction.
  - The use of nitrates for the treatment of coronary artery disease or to modify hemodynamics.
- The Examiner must defer issuance of a medical certificate to any applicant whose hypertension has not been evaluated, who uses unacceptable medications, whose medical status is unclear, whose hypertension is uncontrolled, who manifests significant adverse effects of medication, or whose certification has previously been specifically reserved to the FAA.

III. Aerospace Medical Disposition

The following is a table that lists the most common conditions of aeromedical significance, and course of action that should be taken by the examiner as defined by the protocol and disposition in the table. Medical certificates must not be issued to an applicant with medical conditions that require deferral, or for any condition not listed in the table that may result in sudden or subtle incapacitation without consulting the AMCD or the RFS. Medical documentation must be submitted for any condition in order to support an issuance of an airman medical certificate.

DISEASE/CONDITION	CLASS	EVALUATION DATA	DISPOSITION
Arrhythmias			
Bradycardia (<50 bpm)	All	Document history and findings, CVE Protocol, and submit any tests deemed appropriate	If no evidence of structural, functional or coronary heart disease - Issue Otherwise - Requires FAA Decision
Bundle Branch Block (Left and Right)	All	See CVE and GXT Protocols See GXT Additional BBB Requirements	If no evidence of structural, functional or coronary heart disease - Issue Otherwise - Requires FAA Decision
History of Implanted Pacemakers	All	See Implanted Pacemaker Protocol	Requires FAA Decision
PAC (2 or more on ECG)	All	Requires evaluation, e.g., check for MVP, caffeine, pulmonary disease, thyroid, etc.	If no evidence of structural, functional or coronary heart disease - Issue Otherwise - Requires FAA Decision
PVC's (2 or more on standard ECG)	All	Max GXT – to include a baseline ECG	If no evidence of structural, functional or coronary heart disease and PVC's resolve with exercise - Issue Otherwise - Requires FAA Decision

DISEASE/CONDITION	CLASS	EVALUATION DATA	DISPOSITION
Arrhythmias			
1st Degree AV Block	All	Document history and findings, CVE Protocol, and submit any tests deemed appropriate	If no evidence of structural, functional or coronary heart disease - Issue Otherwise - Requires FAA Decision
2nd Degree AV Block Mobitz I	All	Document history and findings, CVE Protocol, and submit any tests deemed appropriate	If no evidence of structural, functional or coronary heart disease - Issue Otherwise - Requires FAA Decision
2nd Degree AV Block Mobitz II	All	CVE Protocol in accordance w/ Hypertensive Evaluation Specifications and 24-hour Holter	Requires FAA Decision
3rd Degree AV Block	All	CVE Protocol in accordance w/ Hypertensive Evaluation Specifications and 24-hour Holter	Requires FAA Decision
Preexcitation	All	CVE Protocol, GXT, and 24-hour Holter	Requires FAA Decision
Radio Frequency Ablation	All	3-month wait, then 24-hour Holter	If Holter negative for arrhythmia and no recurrence – Issue Otherwise - Requires FAA Decision

DISEASE/CONDITION	CLASS	EVALUATION DATA	DISPOSITION
Arrhythmias			
Supraventricular Tachycardia	All	CHD Protocol with ECHO and 24-hour Holter	**Initial Special Issuance** - Requires FAA Decision **Followup Special Issuance's** - See AASI Protocol
Atrial Fibrillation			
Atrial Fibrillation: Chronic Paroxysmal/Lone	All	CVE Protocol with EST, ECHO and 24-hour Holter.	**Initial Special Issuance** - Requires FAA Decision **Followup Special Issuance's** - See AASI Protocol
History of Resolved Atrial Fibrillation >5 years ago	All	Document previous workup for CAD and structural heart disease	If no ischemia, history of emboli, or structural or functional heart disease - Issue Otherwise - Requires FAA Decision
Coronary Heart Disease			
Coronary Heart Disease: Angina Pectoris Atherectomy;	1st & 2nd	See CHD Protocol	Requires FAA Decision
Coronary Bypass Grafting; Myocardial Infarction; PTCA; Rotoblation; and Stent Insertion	3rd	See CHD Protocol	**Initial Special Issuance** - Requires FAA Decision **Followup Special Issuance's** - See AASI Protocol

Hypertension			
Hypertension requiring medication		See Hypertension Protocol	If controlled on acceptable medication and no complications – Issue Otherwise - Requires FAA Decision
Syncope			
Syncope	All	CHD Protocol with ECHO and 24-hour Holter; bilatcarotid Ultrasound	Requires FAA Decision Syncope, recurrent or not satisfactorily explained, requires deferral (even though the syncope episode may be medically explained, an aeromedical certification decision may still be precluded). Syncope may involve cardiovascular, neurological, and psychiatric factors.
Valvular Disease			
All Other Valvular Disease	All	CHD Protocol with ECHO	Requires FAA Decision
Aortic and Mitral Insufficiency	All	CHD Protocol with ECHO	**Initial Special Issuance** - Requires FAA Decision **Followup Special Issuance's** - See AASI Protocol
Single Valve Replacement (Tissue, Mechanical or Valvuloplasty)	1st & 2nd	See Cardiac Valve Replacement	Requires FAA Decision
	3rd		**Initial Special Issuance** - Requires FAA Decision **Followup Special Issuance's** - See AASI Protocol
Multiple Valve Replacement	All	Document history and findings, CVE Protocol, and submit appropriate tests.	Requires FAA Decision

Other Cardiac Conditions

The following conditions must be deferred:

1. Cardiac Transplant – see Disease Protocols.
2. Cardiac decompensation.
3. Congenital heart disease accompanied by cardiac enlargement, ECG abnormality, or evidence of inadequate oxygenation.
4. Hypertrophy or dilatation of the heart as evidenced by clinical examination and supported by diagnostic studies.
5. Pericarditis, endocarditis, or myocarditis.
6. When cardiac enlargement or other evidence of cardiovascular abnormality is found, the decision is deferred to AMCD or RFS. If the applicant wishes further consideration, a consultation will be required "preferably" from the applicant's treating physician. It must include a narrative report of evaluation and be accompanied by an ECG with report and appropriate laboratory test results which may include, as appropriate, 24-hour Holter monitoring, thyroid function studies, ECHO, and an assessment of coronary artery status. The report and accompanying materials should be forwarded to the AMCD or RFS.
7. Anti-tachycardia devices or implantable defibrillators.
8. With the possible exceptions of aspirin and dipyridamole taken for their effect on blood platelets, the use of anticoagulants or other drugs for treatment or prophylaxis of fibrillation may preclude medical certification.
9. A history of cardioversion or drug treatment, *per se,* does not rule out certification. A current, complete cardiovascular evaluation will be required. A 3-month observation period must elapse after the procedure before consideration for certification.
10. Any other cardiac disorder not otherwise covered in this section.
11. For all classes, certification decisions will be based on the applicant's medical history and current clinical findings. Certification is unlikely unless the information is highly favorable to the applicant. Evidence of extensive multi-vessel disease, impaired cardiac functioning, precarious coronary circulation, etc., will preclude certification. Before an applicant undergoes coronary angiography, it is recommended that all records and the report of a current cardiovascular evaluation, including a maximal electrocardiographic exercise stress test, be submitted to the FAA for preliminary review. Based upon this information, it may be possible to advise an applicant of the likelihood of favorable consideration.
12. A history of low blood pressure requires elaboration. If the Examiner is in doubt, it is usually better to defer issuance rather than to deny certification for such a history.

ITEM 37. Vascular System

CHECK EACH ITEM IN APPROPRIATE COLUMN	Normal	Abnormal
37. Vascular System		

I. Code of Federal Regulations

All Classes: 14 CFR 67.113(b)(c), 67.213(b)(c), and 67.313(b)(c)

(b) No other organic, functional, or structural disease, defect, or limitation that the Federal Air Surgeon, based on the case history and appropriate, qualified medical judgment relating to the condition involved, finds –

    (1) Makes the person unable to safely perform the duties or exercise the privileges of the airman certificate applied for or held; or

    (2) May reasonably be expected, for the maximum duration of the airman medical certificate applied for or held, to make the person unable to perform those duties or exercise those privileges;

(c) No medication or other treatment that the Federal Air Surgeon, based on the case history and appropriate, qualified medical judgment relating to the medication or other treatment involved, finds -

    (1) Makes the person unable to safely perform the duties or exercise the privileges of the airman certificate applied for or held; or

    (2) May reasonably be expected, for the maximum duration of the airman medical certificate applied for or held, to make the person unable to perform those duties or exercise those privileges.

II. Examination Techniques

1. Inspection. Observe and report any thoracic deformity (e.g., pectus excavatum), signs of surgery or other trauma, and clues to ventricular hypertrophy. Check the hematopoietic and vascular system by observing for pallor, edema, varicosities, stasis ulcers, venous distention, nail beds for capillary pulsation, and color.

2. Palpation. Check for thrills and the vascular system for arteriosclerotic changes, shunts or AV anastomoses. The pulses should be examined to determine their character, to note if they are diminished or absent, and to observe for synchronicity.

3. Percussion. N/A.

4. Auscultation. Check for bruits and thrills.

III. Aerospace Medical Disposition

The following is a table that lists the most common conditions of aeromedical significance, and course of action that should be taken by the examiner as defined by the protocol and disposition in the table. Medical certificates must not be issued to an applicant with medical conditions that require deferral, or for any condition not listed in the table that may result in sudden or subtle incapacitation without consulting the AMCD or the RFS. Medical documentation must be submitted for any condition in order to support an issuance of an airman medical certificate.

DISEASE/CONDITION	CLASS	EVALUATION DATA	DISPOSITION
Vascular Conditions			
Aneurysm (Abdominal or Thoracic)	All	Submit all available medical documentation	Requires FAA Decision
Aneurysm (Status Post Repair)	All	Submit all documentation in accordance with CVE Protocol, and include a GXT	Requires FAA Decision
Arteriosclerotic Vascular disease with evidence of circulatory obstruction	All	Submit all documentation in accordance with CVE Protocol, and include a GXT, and CAD ultra sound if applicable	Requires FAA Decision
Buerger's Disease	All	Document history and findings	If no impairment and no symptoms in flight - Issue Otherwise - Requires FAA Decision

DISEASE/CONDITION	CLASS	EVALUATION DATA	DISPOSITION
Vascular Conditions			
Peripheral Edema	All	The underlying medical condition must not be disqualifying	If findings can be explained by normal physiologic response or secondary to medication(s) - Issue Otherwise - Requires FAA Decision
Raynaud's Disease	All	Document history and findings	If no impairment - Issue Otherwise - Requires FAA Decision
Phlebothrombosis or Thrombophlebitis	1st & 2nd	See Thrombophlebitis Protocol	Requires FAA Decision
	3rd	Document history and findings	A single episode resolved, not currently treated with anticoagulants, and a negative evaluation - Issue
		See Thrombophlebitis Protocol	If history of multiple episodes - Requires FAA Decision

ITEM 38. Abdomen and Viscera

CHECK EACH ITEM IN APPROPRIATE COLUMN	Normal	Abnormal
38. Abdomen and viscera (including hernia)		

I. Code of Federal Regulations

All Classes: 14 CFR 67.113(b)(c), 67.213(b)(c), and 67.313(b)(c)

(b) No other organic, functional, or structural disease, defect, or limitation that the Federal Air Surgeon, based on the case history and appropriate, qualified medical judgment relating to the medication or other treatment involved, finds-

    (1) Makes the person unable to safely perform the duties or exercise the privileges of the airman certificate applied for or held; or

    (2) May reasonably be expected, for the maximum duration of the airman medical certificate applied for or held, to make the person unable to perform those duties or exercise those privileges.

(c) No medication or other treatment that the Federal Air Surgeon, based on the case history and appropriate, qualified medical judgment relating to the medication or other treatment involved, finds -

    (1) Makes the person unable to safely perform the duties or exercise the privileges of the airman certificate applied for or held; or

    (2) May reasonably be expected, for the maximum duration of the airman medical certificate applied for or held, to make the person unable to perform those duties or exercise those privileges.

II. Examination Techniques

1. Observation: The Examiner should note any unusual shape or contour, skin color, moisture, temperature, and presence of scars. Hernias, hemorrhoids, and fissure should be noted and recorded.

A history of acute gastrointestinal disorders is usually not disqualifying once recovery is achieved, e.g., acute appendicitis.

Many chronic gastrointestinal diseases may preclude issuance of a medical certificate (e.g., cirrhosis, chronic hepatitis, malignancy, ulcerative colitis). Colostomy following surgery for cancer may be allowed by the FAA with special followup reports.

The Examiner should not issue a medical certificate if the applicant has a recent history of bleeding ulcers or hemorrhagic colitis. Otherwise, ulcers must not have been active within the past 3 months.

In the case of a history of bowel obstruction, a report on the cause and present status of the condition must be obtained from the treating physician.

2. Palpation: The Examiner should check for and note enlargement of organs, unexplained masses, tenderness, guarding, and rigidity.

III. Aerospace Medical Disposition

The following is a table that lists the most common conditions of aeromedical significance, and course of action that should be taken by the examiner as defined by the protocol and disposition in the table. Medical certificates must not be issued to an applicant with medical conditions that require deferral, or for any condition not listed in the table that may result in sudden or subtle incapacitation without consulting the AMCD or the RFS. Medical documentation must be submitted for any condition in order to support an issuance of an airman medical certificate.

DISEASE/CONDITION	CLASS	EVALUATION DATA	DISPOSITION
Abdomen and Viscera and Anus Conditions			
Cholelithiasis	All	Document history and findings	If asymptomatic - Issue Otherwise - Requires FAA Decision
Cirrhosis (Alcoholic)	All	See Substance Abuse/Dependence Disposition in Item 47.	Requires FAA Decision
Cirrhosis (Non-Alcoholic)	All	Submit all pertinent medical records, current status report, to include history of encephalopathy; PT/PTT; albumin; liver enzymes; bilirubin; CBC; and other testing deemed necessary	Requires FAA Decision

DISEASE/CONDITION	CLASS	EVALUATION DATA	DISPOSITION
Abdomen and Viscera and Anus Conditions			
Colitis (Ulcerative, Regional Enteritis or Crohn's disease)	All	Submit all pertinent medical information and current status report, include duration of symptoms, name and dosage of drugs and side effects	**Initial Special Issuance** - Requires FAA Decision **Followup Special Issuance's** - See AASI Protocol
Hepatitis	All	Submit all pertinent medical records, current status report to include any other testing deemed necessary	If disease is resolved without sequela - Issue Otherwise - Requires FAA Decision
Hepatitis C	All	Submit all pertinent medical information and current status report, include duration of symptoms, name and dosage of drugs and side effects	**Initial Special Issuance** - Requires FAA Decision **Followup Special Issuance's** - See AASI Protocol
Inguinal, Ventral or Hiatal Hernia	All	Document history and findings	If symptomatic; likely to cause any degree of obstruction - Requires FAA Decision Otherwise - Issue
Liver Transplant	All	Submit all pertinent medical information and current status report, include duration of symptoms, name and dosage of drugs and side effects	Requires FAA Decision
Peptic Ulcer	All	See Peptic Ulcer Protocol	Requires FAA Decision
Splenomegaly	All	Provide hematologic workup	Requires FAA Decision

DISEASE/CONDITION	CLASS	EVALUATION DATA	DISPOSITION
Malignancies			
Colon/Rectal Cancer	All	Submit all pertinent medical records, operative/ pathology reports, current oncological status report; and current CEA and CBC	**Initial Special Issuance** - Requires FAA Decision **Followup Special Issuance's** - See AASI Protocol
Other Malignances	All	Submit all pertinent medical records, operative/ pathology reports, current oncological status report, including tumor markers, and any other testing deemed necessary	Requires FAA Decision

An applicant with an ileostomy or colostomy may also receive FAA consideration. A report is necessary to confirm that the applicant has fully recovered from the surgery and is completely asymptomatic.

In the case of a history of bowel obstruction, a report on the cause and present status of the condition must be obtained from the treating physician.

ITEM 39. Anus

CHECK EACH ITEM IN APPROPRIATE COLUMN	Normal	Abnormal
39 Anus (Not including digital examination)		

I. Code of Federal Regulations

All Classes: 14 CFR 67.113(a), 67.213(b)(c), and 67.313(b)(c)

(b) No other organic, functional, or structural disease, defect, or limitation that the Federal Air Surgeon, based on the case history and appropriate, qualified medical judgment relating to the medication or other treatment involved, finds

(1) Makes the person unable to safely perform the duties or exercise the privileges of the airman certificate applied for or held; or

(2) May reasonably be expected, for the maximum duration of the airman medical certificate applied for or held, to make the person unable to perform those duties or exercise those privileges.

(c) No medication or other treatment that the Federal Air Surgeon, based on the case history and appropriate, qualified medical judgment relating to the medication or other treatment involved, finds -

(1) Makes the person unable to safely perform the duties or exercise the privileges of the airman certificate applied for or held; or

(2) May reasonably be expected, for the maximum duration of the airman medical certificate applied for or held, to make the person unable to perform those duties or exercise those privileges.

II. Examination Techniques

1. Digital Rectal Examination: This examination is performed only at the applicant's option unless indicated by specific history or physical findings. When performed, the following should be noted and recorded in Item 59 of FAA Form 8500-8.

2. If the digital rectal examination is not performed, the response to Item 39 may be based on direct observation or history.

ITEM 40. Skin

CHECK EACH ITEM IN APPROPRIATE COLUMN	NORMAL	ABNORMAL
40. Skin		

I. Code of Federal Regulations

All Classes: 14 CFR 67.113(b)(c), 67.213(b)(c), and 67.313(b)(c)

(b) No other organic, functional, or structural disease, defect, or limitation that the Federal Air Surgeon, based on the case history and appropriate, qualified medical judgment relating to the condition involved, finds -

(1) Makes the person unable to safely perform the duties or exercise the privileges of the airman certificate applied for or held; or

(2) May reasonably be expected, for the maximum duration of the airman medical certificate applied for or held, to make the person unable to perform those duties or exercise those privileges.

(c) No medication or other treatment that the Federal Air Surgeon, based on the case history and appropriate, qualified medical judgment relating to the medication or other treatment involved, finds -

    (1) Makes the person unable to safely perform the duties or exercise the privileges of the airman certificate applied for or held; or

    (2) May reasonably be expected, for the maximum duration of the airman medical certificate applied for or held, to make the person unable to perform those duties or exercise those privileges.

II. Examination Techniques

A careful examination of the skin may reveal underlying systemic disorders of clinical importance. For example, thyroid disease may produce changes in the skin and fingernails. Cushing's disease may produce abdominal striae, and abnormal pigmentation of the skin occurs with Addison's disease.

Needle marks that suggest drug abuse should be noted and body marks and scars should be described and correlated with known history. Further history should be obtained as needed to explain findings.

The use of isotretinoin (Accutane) can be associated with vision and psychiatric side effects of aeromedical concern – specifically decreased night vision/night blindness and depression. These side-effects can occur even after the cessation of isotretinoin. See Aeromedical Decision Considerations.

III. Aerospace Medical Disposition

The following is a table that lists the most common conditions of aeromedical significance, and course of action that should be taken by the examiner as defined by the protocol and disposition in the table. Medical certificates must not be issued to an applicant with medical conditions that require deferral, or for any condition not listed in the table that may result in sudden or subtle incapacitation without consulting the AMCD or the RFS. Medical documentation must be submitted for any condition in order to support an issuance of an airman medical certificate.

DISEASE/CONDITION	CLASS	EVALUATION DATA	DISPOSITION
Cutaneous			
Dermatomyositis; Deep Mycotic Infections; Eruptive Xanthomas; Hansen's Disease; Lupus Erythematosus; Raynaud's Phenomenon; Sarcoid; or Scleroderma	All	Submit all pertinent medical information and current status report	Requires FAA Decision
Kaposi's Sarcoma	All	Submit all pertinent medical information and current status report. See HIV Protocol	Requires FAA Decision

DISEASE/CONDITION	CLASS	EVALUATION DATA	DISPOSITION
Cutaneous			
Use of isotretinoin (Accutane)	All	For applicants using isotretinoin, there is a mandatory 2-week waiting period after starting isotretinoin prior to consideration. This medication can be associated with vision and psychiatric side effects of aeromedical concern - specifically decreased night vision/night blindness and depression. These side-effects can occur even after cessation of isotretinoin. A report must be provided with detailed, specific comment on presence or absence of psychiatric and vision side-effects. The AME must document these findings in Item 60., Comments on History and Findings.	Any history of psychiatric side-effect requires FAA Decision. If there are no vision, psychiatric, or other aeromedically unacceptable side-effects – Issue with restriction: "NOT VALID FOR NIGHT FLYING." To remove restriction: *See Note

*Note:
- Use of isotretinoin must be permanently discontinued for at least 2 weeks prior to consideration date (confirmed by the prescribing physician)
- An eye evaluation in accordance with specifications in 8500-7
- Airman must provide a statement of discontinuation
  - Confirming the absence of any visual disturbances and psychiatric symptoms, and
  - Acknowledging requirement to notify the FAA and obtain clearance prior to performing any aviation safety-related duties if use of isotretinoin is resumed

DISEASE/CONDITION	CLASS	EVALUATION DATA	DISPOSITION
Malignant Melanoma			
Melanoma Level >.75 mm with/ without any metastasis	All	Submit all pertinent medical records, operative/ pathology reports, and current oncological status report, and current MRI of the brain	**Initial Special Issuance** - Requires FAA Decision **Followup Special Issuance's** - See AASI Protocol
Melanoma of Unknown Primary Origin	All	Submit all pertinent medical records, operative/ pathology reports, and current oncological status report, current MRI of the brain; PET scan if no primary	Requires FAA Decision
Urticarial Eruptions			
Angioneurotic Edema	All	Submit all pertinent medical records and a current status report to include treatment	Requires FAA Decision
Chronic Urticaria	All	Submit all records and a current status report to include treatment	Requires FAA Decision

ITEM 41. G-U System

CHECK EACH ITEM IN APPROPRIATE COLUMN	NORMAL	ABNORMAL
41. G-U system (Not including pelvic examination)		

NOTE: The pelvic examination is performed only at the applicant's option or if indicated by specific history or physical findings. If a pelvic examination is performed, the results are to be recorded in Item 60 of FAA Form 8500-8.

I. Code of Federal Regulations

All Classes: 14 CFR 67.113(b)(c), 67.213(b)(c), and 67.313(b)(c)

(b) No other organic, functional, or structural disease, defect, or limitation that the Federal Air Surgeon, based on the case history and appropriate, qualified medical judgment relating to the condition involved, finds -

(1) Makes the person unable to safely perform the duties or exercise the privileges of the airman certificate applied for or held; or

(2) May reasonably be expected, for the maximum duration of the airman medical certificate applied for or held, to make the person unable to perform those duties or exercise those privileges.

(c) No medication or other treatment that the Federal Air Surgeon, based on the case history and appropriate, qualified medical judgment relating to the medication or other treatment involved, finds -

(1) Makes the person unable to safely perform the duties or exercise the privileges of the airman certificate applied for or held; or

(2) May reasonably be expected, for the maximum duration of the airman medical certificate applied for or held, to make the person unable to perform those duties or exercise those privileges.

II. Examination Techniques

The Examiner should observe for discharge, inflammation, skin lesions, scars, strictures, tumors, and secondary sexual characteristics. Palpation for masses and areas of tenderness should be performed. The pelvic examination is performed only at the applicant's option or if indicated by specific history or physical findings. If a pelvic examination is performed, the results are to be recorded in Item 60 of FAA Form 8500-8. Disorders such as sterility and menstrual irregularity are not usually of importance in qualification for medical certification.

Specialty evaluations may be indicated by history or by physical findings on the routine examination. A personal history of urinary symptoms is important; such as:

1. Pain or burning upon urination

2. Dribbling or Incontinence

3. Polyuria, frequency, or nocturia

4. Hematuria, pyuria, or glycosuria

Special procedures for evaluation of the G-U system should best be left to the discretion of an urologist, nephrologist, or gynecologist.

III. Aerospace Medical Disposition

(See **Item 48., General Systemic**, for details concerning diabetes and **Item 57., Urine Test**, for other information related to the examination of urine).

The following is a table that lists the most common conditions of aeromedical significance, and course of action that should be taken by the examiner as defined by the protocol and disposition in the table. Medical certificates must not be issued to an applicant with medical conditions that require deferral, or for any condition not listed in the table that may result in sudden or subtle incapacitation without consulting the AMCD or the RFS. Medical documentation must be submitted for any condition in order to support an issuance of an airman medical certificate.

DISEASE/CONDITION	CLASS	EVALUATION DATA	DISPOSITION
General Disorders			
Congenital lesions of the kidney	All	Submit all pertinent medical information and status report	If the applicant has an ectopic, horseshoe kidney, unilateral agenesis, hypoplastic, or dysplastic and is asymptomatic – Issue Otherwise – Requires FAA Decision

DISEASE/CONDITION	CLASS	EVALUATION DATA	DISPOSITION
General Disorders			
Cystostomy and Neurogenic bladder	All	Requires evaluation, report must include etiology, clinical manifestation and treatment plan	Requires FAA Decision
Renal Dialysis	All	Submit a current status report, all pertinent medical reports to include etiology, clinical manifestation, BUN, Ca, PO^4, Creatinine, electrolytes, and treatment plan	Requires FAA Decision
Renal Transplant	All	See **Renal Transplant Protocol**	Requires FAA Decision
Inflammatory Conditions			
Acute (Nephritis)	All	Submit all pertinent medical information and status report	If > 3 mos. ago, resolved, no sequela, or indication of reoccurrence - Issue Otherwise - Requires FAA Decision
Chronic (Nephritis)	All	Submit all pertinent medical information and status report	Requires FAA Decision
Nephrosis	All	Submit all pertinent medical information and status report	Requires FAA Decision

DISEASE/CONDITION	CLASS	EVALUATION DATA	DISPOSITION
Neoplastic Disorders			
Bladder	All	Submit all pertinent medical records, operative/ pathology reports, current oncological status report, including tumor markers, and any other testing deemed necessary report, include duration of symptoms, name and dosage of drugs and side effects	**Initial Special Issuance** - Requires FAA Decision **Followup Special Issuance's** - See AASI Protocol
Other Neoplastic Disorders	All	Submit a current status report, all pertinent medical reports to include staging, metastatic work up, and operative report if applicable	Requires FAA Decision
Prostatic Cancer	All	Submit a current status report, all pertinent medical reports to include staging, PSA, metastatic workup, and operative report, if applicable, and treatment	**Initial Special Issuance** - Requires FAA Decision **Followup Special Issuance's** - See AASI Protocol

DISEASE/CONDITION	CLASS	EVALUATION DATA	DISPOSITION
Neoplastic Disorders			
Renal Carcinoma	All	Submit all pertinent medical records, operative/ pathology reports, current oncological status report, including tumor markers, and any other testing deemed necessary report, include duration of symptoms, name and dosage of drugs and side effects	**Initial Special Issuance** - Requires FAA Decision **Followup Special Issuance's** - See AASI Protocol
Testicular Carcinoma	All	Submit all pertinent medical records, operative/ pathology reports, current oncological status report, and any other testing deemed necessary report, include duration of symptoms, name and dosage of drugs and side effects	**Initial Special Issuance** - Requires FAA Decision **Followup Special Issuance's** - See AASI Protocol
Nephritis			
Polycystic Kidney Disease	All	Submit all pertinent medical information and status report	If renal function is normal and no hypertension - Issue Otherwise - Requires FAA Decision
Pyelitis or Pyelonephritis	All	Submit all pertinent medical information and status report	If asymptomatic - Issue Otherwise - Requires FAA Decision

DISEASE/CONDITION	CLASS	EVALUATION DATA	DISPOSITION
Nephritis			
Pyonephrosis	All	Submit all pertinent medical information and status report	Requires FAA Decision
Urinary System			
Hydronephrosis with impaired renal function	All	Submit all pertinent medical information and status report	Requires FAA Decision
Nephrectomy (non-neoplastic)	All	Submit all pertinent medical information and status report	If the remaining kidney function and anatomy is normal, without other systemic disease, hypertension, uremia, infection of the remaining kidney – Issue Otherwise - Requires FAA Decision
Nephrocalcinosis	All	Submit all pertinent medical information and status report	If calculus is not in collecting system or renal pelvis - Issue Otherwise - Requires FAA Decision
Calculus [1] Renal - Single episode	All	Submit current metabolic evaluation and status report	If there is no residual calculi and the metabolic workup is negative - Issue Otherwise - Requires FAA Decision

[1] Complete studies to determine the possible etiology and prognosis are essential to favorable FAA consideration. Determining factors include site and location of the stones, complications such as compromise in renal function, repeated bouts of kidney infection, and need for therapy. Any underlying disease will be considered. The likelihood of sudden incapacitating symptoms is of primary concern. Report of imaging studies (KUB, IVP, or spiral CT) must be submitted in order to conclude that there are no residual or retained calculi.

DISEASE/CONDITION	CLASS	EVALUATION DATA	DISPOSITION
Urinary System			
Renal – Multiple episodes or Retained Stones	All	Submit current metabolic evaluation and status report	**Initial Special Issuance** - Requires FAA Decision **Followup Special Issuance's** - See AASI Protocol
Ureteral or Vesical	All	Single episode and no retained calculi, submit current metabolic evaluation and status report (Ureteral stent is acceptable if functioning without sequela)	If metabolic workup is negative and there is no sequela or retained calculi - Issue Otherwise - Requires FAA Decision

A history of recent or significant hematuria requires further evaluation.

PREGNANCY

Pregnancy under normal circumstances is not disqualifying. It is recommended that the applicant's obstetrician be made aware of all aviation activities so that the obstetrician can properly advise the applicant. The Examiner may wish to counsel applicants concerning piloting aircraft during the third trimester. The proper use of lap belt and shoulder harness warrants discussion.

GENDER IDENTITY DISORDER

Gender Identity Disorder (GID) and gender reassignment require a complete review of the individual's relevant medical history and records. For initial consideration the Examiner must defer and submit the following to AMCD or RFS:

- A current status report to include:
    - All current medications, dosages, and side-effects; and
    - Copies of all pertinent inpatient and outpatient medical records pertaining to the individual's GID diagnosis, work-up, and treatment.

- Psychiatric and/or psychological evaluations by a board certified psychiatrist and/or a licensed psychologist experienced in transgender issues that includes an assessment of any substance abuse or misuse. Neurocognitive testing is not required unless clinically indicated.

- Hospital and post-operative report from the surgeon if individual has had surgery.

NOTE: If the individual refrains from surgery, no surgical report is required. However, if surgery is elected at a later date, follow-up reports from a psychiatrist and/or psychologist and the surgeon will be required.

ITEMS 42-43. Musculoskeletal

CHECK EACH ITEM IN APPROPRIATE COLUMN	NORMAL	ABNORMAL
42. Upper and lower extremities (Strength and range of motion)		
43. Spine, other musculoskeletal		

I. Code of Federal Regulations

All Classes: 14 CFR 67.113 (b)(c), 67.213 (b)(c), and 67.313 (b)(c)

(b) No other organic, functional, or structural disease, defect, or limitation that the Federal Air Surgeon, based on the case history and appropriate, qualified medical judgment relating to the condition involved finds -

(1) Makes the person unable to safely perform the duties or exercise the privileges of the airman certificate applied for or held; or

(2) May reasonably be expected, for the maximum duration of the airman medical certificate applied for or held, to make the person unable to perform those duties or exercise those privileges.

(c) No medication or other treatment that the Federal Air Surgeon, based on the case history and appropriate, qualified medical judgment relating to the medication or other treatment involved, finds -

(1) Makes the person unable to safely perform the duties or exercise the privileges of the airman certificate applied for or held; or

(2) May reasonably be expected, for the maximum duration of the   airman medical certificate applied for or held, to make the person unable to perform those duties or exercise those privileges.

II. Examination Techniques

Standard examination procedures should be used to make a gross evaluation of the integrity of the applicant's musculoskeletal system. The Examiner should note:

1. Pain - neuralgia, myalgia, paresthesia, and related circulatory and neurological findings

2. Weakness - local or generalized; degree and amount of functional loss

3. Paralysis - atrophy, contractures, and related dysfunctions

4. Motion coordination, tremors, loss or restriction of joint motions, and performance degradation

5. Deformity - extent and cause

6. Amputation - level, stump healing, and phantom pain

7. Prostheses - comfort and ability to use effectively

III. Aerospace Medical Disposition

The following is a table that lists the most common conditions of aeromedical significance, and course of action that should be taken by the examiner as defined by the protocol and disposition in the table. Medical certificates must not be issued to an applicant with medical conditions that require deferral, or for any condition not listed in the table that may result in sudden or subtle incapacitation without consulting the AMCD or the RFS. Medical documentation must be submitted for any condition in order to support an issuance of an airman medical certificate.

ITEM 42. Upper and Lower Extremities

DISEASE/CONDITION	CLASS	EVALUATION DATA	DISPOSITION
Upper and Lower Extremities			
Amputations	All	Submit a current status report to include functional status (degree of impairment as measured by strength, range of motion, pain), medications with side effects and all pertinent medical reports	If applicant has a SODA issued on the basis of the amputation - Issue Otherwise - Requires FAA Decision After review of all medical data, the FAA may authorize a special medical flight test
Atrophy of any muscles that is progressive, Deformities, either congenital or acquired, or Limitation of motion of a major joint, that are sufficient to interfere with the performance of airman duties	All	Submit a current status report to include functional status (degree of impairment as measured by strength, range of motion, pain), medication with side effects, and all pertinent medical reports	Requires FAA Decision

DISEASE/CONDITION	CLASS	EVALUATION DATA	DISPOSITION
Upper and Lower Extremities			
Neuralgia or Neuropathy, chronic or acute, particularly sciatica, if sufficient to interfere with function or is likely to become incapacitating	All	Submit a current status report to include functional status (degree of impairment as measured by strength, range of motion, pain), medications with side effects and all pertinent medical reports	Requires FAA Decision
Osteomyelitis, acute or chronic, with or without draining fistula(e)	All	Submit a current status report to include functional status (degree of impairment as measured by strength, range of motion, pain), medications with side effects and all pertinent medical reports	Requires FAA Decision
Tremors, if sufficient to interfere with the performance of airman duties[1]	All	Submit a current status report to include functional status (degree of impairment as measured by strength, range of motion, pain), medications with side effects and all pertinent medical reports	Requires FAA Decision

---

[1] Essential tremor is not disqualifying unless it is disabling.

For all the above conditions: If the applicant is otherwise qualified, the FAA may issue a limited certificate. This certificate will permit the applicant to proceed with flight training until ready for a MFT. At that time, at the applicant's request, the FAA (usually the AMCD) will authorize the student pilot to take a MFT in conjunction with the regular flight test. The MFT and regular private pilot flight test are conducted by an FAA inspector. This affords the student an opportunity to demonstrate the ability to control the aircraft despite the handicap. The FAA inspector prepares a written report and indicates whether there is a safety problem. A medical certificate and SODA, without the student limitation, may be provided to the inspector for issuance to the applicant, or the inspector may be required to send the report to the FAA medical officer who authorized the test.

When prostheses are used or additional control devices are installed in an aircraft to assist the amputee, those found qualified by special certification procedures will have their certificates limited to require that the devices (and, if necessary, even the specific aircraft) must always be used when exercising the privileges of the airman certificate.

Item 43. Spine, Other Musculoskeletal

DISEASE/CONDITION	CLASS	EVALUATION DATA	DISPOSITION
Arthritis			
Osteoarthritis [1]	All	Submit a current status report to include functional status (degree of impairment as measured by strength, range of motion, pain), medications with side effects and all pertinent medical reports	If mild and controlled with small doses of nonprescription agents - Issue If symptomatic or requires medication - Requires FAA Decision

---

[1] Arthritis (if it is symptomatic or requires medication, other than small doses of nonprescription anti-inflammatory agents), is disqualifying unless the applicant holds a letter from the FAA specifically authorizing the Examiner to issue the certificate when the applicant is found otherwise qualified. Although the use of many medications on a continuing basis ordinarily contraindicates the performance of pilot duties, under certain circumstances, certification is possible for an applicant who is taking aspirin, ibuprofen, naproxen, similar nonsteroidal anti-inflammatory drugs (NSAID), or COX-2 inhibitors. If the applicant presents evidence documenting that the underlying condition for which the medicine is being taken is not in itself disabling and the applicant has been on therapy (NSAID) long enough to have established that the medication is well tolerated and has not produced adverse side effects, the Examiner may issue a certificate.

DISEASE/CONDITION	CLASS	EVALUATION DATA	DISPOSITION
Arthritis			
Rheumatoid Arthritis and Variants	All	Submit a current status report to include functional status (degree of impairment as measured by strength, range of motion, pain), medications with side effects and all pertinent medical reports	**Initial Special Issuance** - Requires FAA Decision **Followup Special Issuance's** - See AASI Protocol
Collagen Disease			
Acute Polymyositis; Dermatomyositis; Lupus Erythematosus; or Periarteritis Nodosa	All	Submit a current status report to include functional status, frequency and severity of episodes, organ systems effected, medications with side effects and all pertinent medical reports	Requires FAA Decision

DISEASE/CONDITION	CLASS	EVALUATION DATA	DISPOSITION
Spine, other musculoskeletal			
Active disease of bones and joints	All	Submit a current status report to include functional status (degree of impairment as measured by strength, range of motion, pain), medications with side effects and all pertinent medical reports	Requires FAA Decision
Ankylosis, curvature, or other marked deformity of the spinal column sufficient to interfere with the performance of airman duties	All	Submit a current status report to include functional status (degree of impairment as measured by strength, range of motion, pain), medications with side effects and all pertinent medical reports	Requires FAA Decision

DISEASE/CONDITION	CLASS	EVALUATION DATA	DISPOSITION
Spine, other musculoskeletal			
Intervertebral Disc Surgery	All	See Footnote[2]	See Footnote[2]

Musculoskeletal effects of:
  Cerebral Palsy,
  Muscular Dystrophy
  Myasthenia Gravis, or
  Myopathies
	All	Submit a current status report to include functional status (degree of impairment as measured by strength, range of motion, pain), medications with side effects and all pertinent medical reports	Requires FAA Decision

Other disturbances of musculoskeletal function, acquired or congenital, sufficient to interfere with the performance of airman duties or likely to progress to that degree	All	Submit a current status report to include functional status (degree of impairment as measured by strength, range of motion, pain), medications with side effects and all pertinent medical reports	Requires FAA Decision

[2] A history of intervertebral disc surgery is not disqualifying. If the applicant is asymptomatic, has completely recovered from surgery, is taking no medication, and has suffered no neurological deficit, the Examiner should confirm these facts in a brief statement in Item 60. The Examiner may then issue any class of medical certificate, providing that the individual meets all the medical standards for that class.

The paraplegic whose paralysis is not the result of a progressive disease process is considered in much the same manner as an amputee. The Examiner should defer issuance and may advise the applicant to request further FAA consideration. The applicant may be authorized to take a MFT along with the private pilot certificate flight test. If successful, the limitation VALID FOR STUDENT PILOT PURPOSES ONLY is removed from the medical certificate, but operational limitations may be added. A statement of demonstrated ability is issued.

Other neuromuscular conditions are covered in more detail in Item 46.

DISEASE/CONDITION	CLASS	EVALUATION DATA	DISPOSITION
Spine, other musculoskeletal			
Symptomatic herniation of intervertebral disc	All	Submit a current status report to include functional status (degree of impairment as measured by strength, range of motion, pain), medications with side effects and all pertinent medical reports	Requires FAA Decision

ITEM 44. Identifying Body Marks, Scars, Tattoos

CHECK EACH ITEM IN APPROPRIATE COLUMN	NORMAL	ABNORMAL
44. Identifying body marks, scars, tattoos (Size and location)		

I. Code of Federal Regulations

All Classes: 14 CFR 67.113(b), 67.213(b), and 67.313(b)

(b) No other organic, functional, or structural disease, defect, or limitation that the Federal Air Surgeon, based on the case history and appropriate, qualified medical judgment relating to the condition finds-

   (1) Makes the person unable to safely perform the duties or exercise the privileges of the airman certificate applied for or held; or

   (2) May reasonably be expected, for the maximum duration of the airman medical certificate applied for or held, to make the person unable to perform those duties or exercise those privileges

II. Examination Techniques

A careful examination for surgical and other scars should be made, and those that are significant (the result of surgery or that could be useful as identifying marks) should be described. Tattoos should be recorded because they may be useful for identification.

III. Aerospace Medical Disposition

The Examiner should question the applicant about any surgical scars that have not been previously addressed, and document the findings in Item 60 of FAA Form 8500-8. Medical certificates must not be issued to applicants with medical conditions that require deferral without consulting the AMCD or RFS. Medical documentation must be submitted for any condition in order to support an issuance of a medical certificate.

Disqualifying Condition: Scar tissue that involves the loss of function, which may interfere with the safe performance of airman duties.

ITEM 45. Lymphatics

CHECK EACH ITEM IN APPROPRIATE COLUMN	NORMAL	ABNORMAL
45. Lymphatics		

I. Code of Federal Regulations

All Classes: 14 CFR 67.113(b)(c), 67.213(b)(c), and 67.313(b)(c)

(b) No other organic, functional, or structural disease, defect, or limitation that the Federal Air Surgeon, based on the case history and appropriate, qualified medical judgment relating to the condition involved, finds -

    (1) Makes the person unable to safely perform the duties or exercise the privileges of the airman certificate applied for or held; or

    (2) May reasonably be expected, for the maximum duration of the airman medical certificate applied for or held, to make the person unable to perform those duties or exercise those privileges.

(c) No medication or other treatment that the Federal Air Surgeon, based on the case history and appropriate, qualified medical judgment relating to the medication or other treatment involved, finds -

    (1) Makes the person unable to safely perform the duties or exercise the privileges of the airman certificate applied for or held; or

    (2) May reasonably be expected, for the maximum duration of the airman medical certificate applied for or held, to make the person unable to perform those duties or exercise those privileges.

II. Examination Techniques

A careful examination of the lymphatic system may reveal underlying systemic disorders of clinical importance. Further history should be obtained as needed to explain findings.

III. Aerospace Medical Disposition

The following is a table that lists the most common conditions of aeromedical significance, and course of action that should be taken by the examiner as defined by the protocol and disposition in the table. Medical certificates must not be issued to an applicant with medical conditions that require deferral, or for any condition not listed in the table that may result in sudden or subtle incapacitation without consulting the AMCD or the RFS. Medical documentation must be submitted for any condition in order to support an issuance of an airman medical certificate.

DISEASE/CONDITION	CLASS	EVALUATION DATA	DISPOSITION
Lymphoma and Hodgkin's Disease			
Lymphoma and Hodgkin's Disease	All	Submit a current status report and all pertinent medical reports. Include past and present treatment(s).	**Initial Special Issuance** - Requires FAA Decision **Followup Special Issuance's** - See AASI Protocol
Leukemia, Acute and Chronic			
Leukemia, Acute and Chronic – All Types	All	Submit a current status report and all pertinent medical reports	Requires FAA Decision
Chronic Lymphocytic Leukemia	All	Submit a current status report and all pertinent medical reports	**Initial Special Issuance** - Requires FAA Decision **Followup Special Issuance's** - See AASI Protocol

DISEASE/CONDITION	CLASS	EVALUATION DATA	DISPOSITION
Lymphatics			
Adenopathy secondary to Systemic Disease or Metastasis	All	Submit a current status report and all pertinent medical reports	Requires FAA Decision
Lymphedema	All	Submit a current status report and all pertinent medical reports. Note if there are any motion restrictions of the involved extremity	Requires FAA Decision
Lymphosarcoma	All	Submit a current status report and all pertinent medical reports. Include past and present treatment(s).	Requires FAA Decision

ITEM 46. Neurologic

CHECK EACH ITEM IN APPROPRIATE COLUMN	NORMAL	ABNORMAL
46. NEUROLOGIC		

I. Code of Federal Regulations

All Classes: 14 CFR 67.109 (a)(b), 67.209 (a)(b), and 67.309 (a)(b)

(a) No established medical history or clinical diagnosis of any of the following:

(1) Epilepsy

(2) A disturbance of consciousness without satisfactory medical explanation of the cause; or

(3) A transient loss of control of nervous system function(s) without satisfactory medical explanation of the cause;

(b) No other seizure disorder, disturbance of consciousness, or neurologic condition that the Federal Air Surgeon, based on the case history and appropriate, qualified medical judgment relating to the condition involved, finds-

(1) Makes the person unable to safely perform the duties or exercise the privileges of the airman certificate applied for or held; or

(2) May reasonably be expected, for the maximum duration of the airman medical certificate applied for or held, to make the person unable to perform those duties or exercise those privileges.

II. Examination Techniques

A neurologic evaluation should consist of a thorough review of the applicant's history prior to the neurological examination. The Examiner should specifically inquire concerning a history of weakness or paralysis, disturbance of sensation, loss of coordination, or loss of bowel or bladder control. Certain laboratory studies, such as scans and imaging procedures of the head or spine, electroencephalograms, or spinal paracentesis may suggest significant medical history. The Examiner should note conditions identified in Item 60 on the application with facts, such as dates, frequency, and severity of occurrence.

A history of simple headaches without sequela is not disqualifying. Some require only temporary disqualification during periods when the headaches are likely to occur or require treatment. Other types of headaches may preclude certification by the Examiner and require special evaluation and consideration (e.g., migraine and cluster headaches).

One or two episodes of dizziness or even fainting may not be disqualifying. For example, dizziness upon suddenly arising when ill is not a true dysfunction. Likewise, the orthostatic faint associated with moderate anemia is no threat to aviation safety as long as the individual is temporarily disqualified until the anemia is corrected.

An unexplained disturbance of consciousness is disqualifying under the medical standards. Because a disturbance of consciousness may be expected to be totally incapacitating, individuals with such histories pose a high risk to safety and must be denied or deferred by the Examiner. If the cause of the disturbance is explained and a loss of consciousness is not likely to recur, then medical certification may be possible.

The basic neurological examination consists of an examination of the 12 cranial nerves, motor strength, superficial reflexes, deep tendon reflexes, sensation, coordination, mental status, and includes the Babinski reflex and Romberg sign. The Examiner should be aware of any asymmetry in responses because this may be evidence of mild or early abnormalities. The Examiner should evaluate the visual field by direct confrontation or, preferably, by one of the perimetry procedures, especially if there is a suggestion of neurological deficiency.

III. Aerospace Medical Disposition

A history or the presence of any neurological condition or disease that potentially may incapacitate an individual should be regarded as initially disqualifying. Issuance of a medical certificate to an applicant in such cases should be denied or defer, pending further evaluation. A convalescence period following illness or injury may be advisable to permit adequate stabilization of an individual's condition and to reduce the risk of an adverse event. Applications from individuals with potentially disqualifying conditions should be forwarded to the AMCD. Processing such applications can be expedited by including hospital records, consultation reports, and appropriate laboratory and imaging studies, if available. Symptoms or disturbances that are secondary to the underlying condition and that may be acutely incapacitating include pain, weakness, vertigo or in coordination, seizures or a disturbance of consciousness, visual disturbance, or mental confusion. Chronic conditions may be incompatible with safety in aircraft operation because of long-term unpredictability, severe neurologic deficit, or psychological impairment.

The following is a table that lists the most common conditions of aeromedical significance, and course of action that should be taken by the examiner as defined by the protocol and disposition in the table. Medical certificates must not be issued to an applicant with medical conditions that require deferral, or for any condition not listed in the table that may result in sudden or subtle incapacitation without consulting the AMCD or the RFS. Medical documentation must be submitted for any condition in order to support an issuance of an airman medical certificate.

DISEASE/CONDITION	CLASS	EVALUATION DATA	DISPOSITION
Cerebrovascular Disease (including the brain stem) [1]			
Cerebral Thrombosis; Intracerebral or Subarachnoid Hemorrhage Transient Ischemic Attack (TIA);	All	Submit all pertinent medical records, current neurologic report, to include CHD Protocol, Brain MRI, Bilat carotid ultra sound, name and dosage of medication(s) and side effects	Requires FAA Decision

[1] Complete neurological evaluations supplemented with appropriate laboratory and imaging studies are required of applicants with the above conditions. Cerebral arteriography may be necessary for review in cases of subarachnoid hemorrhage.

DISEASE/CONDITION	CLASS	EVALUATION DATA	DISPOSITION
Cerebrovascular Disease			
Intracranial Aneurysm or Arteriovenous Malformation	All	Submit all pertinent medical records, current neurologic report, name and dosage of medication(s) and side effects	Requires FAA Decision
Intracranial Tumor[2]	All	Submit all pertinent medical records, current neurologic report, name and dosage of medication(s) and side effects	Requires FAA Decision
Pseudotumor Cerebri (benign intracranial hypertension)	All	Submit all pertinent medical records, current neurologic report, name and dosage of medication(s) and side effects	Requires FAA Decision

---

[2] A variety of intracranial tumors, both malignant and benign, are capable of causing incapacitation directly by neurologic deficit or indirectly through recurrent symptomatology. Potential neurologic deficits include weakness, loss of sensation, ataxia, visual deficit, or mental impairment. Recurrent symptomatology may interfere with flight performance through mechanisms such as seizure, headaches, vertigo, visual disturbances, or confusion. A history or diagnosis of an intracranial tumor necessitates a complete neurological evaluation with appropriate laboratory and imaging studies before a determination of eligibility for medical certification can be established. An applicant with a history of benign supratentorial tumors may be considered favorably for medical certification by the FAA and returned to flying status after a minimum satisfactory convalescence of 1 year.

DISEASE/CONDITION	CLASS	EVALUATION DATA	DISPOSITION
Demyelinating Disease[3]			
Acute Optic Neuritis; Allergic Encephalomyelitis; Landry-Guillain-Barre Syndrome; Myasthenia Gravis; or Multiple Sclerosis	All	Submit all pertinent medical records, current neurologic report, to comment on involvement and persisting deficit, period of stability without symptoms, name and dosage of medication(s) and side effects	Requires FAA Decision

[3] Factors used in determining eligibility will include the medical history, neurological involvement and persisting deficit, period of stability without symptoms, type and dosage of medications used, and general health. A neurological and/or general medical consultation will be necessary in most instances.

DISEASE/CONDITION	CLASS	EVALUATION DATA	DISPOSITION
Extrapyramidal, Hereditary, and Degenerative Diseases of the Nervous System[4]			
Dystonia Musculorum Deformans; Huntington's Disease; Parkinson's Disease; Wilson's Disease; or Gilles de la Tourette Syndrome; Alzheimer's Disease; Dementia (unspecified); or Slow viral diseases i.e., Creutzfeldt -Jakob's Disease	All	Obtain medical records and current neurological status, complete neurological evaluation with appropriate laboratory and imaging studies, as indicated May consider Neuro-psychological testing	Requires FAA Decision

[4] Extrapyramidal, Hereditary, and Degenerative Diseases of the Nervous System: Considerable variability exists in the severity of involvement, rate of progression, and treatment of the above conditions. A complete neurological evaluation with appropriate laboratory and imaging studies, including information regarding the specific neurological condition, will be necessary for determination of eligibility for medical certification.

DISEASE/CONDITION	CLASS	EVALUATION DATA	DISPOSITION
Headaches[5]			
Atypical Facial Pain	All	Submit all pertinent medical records, current neurologic report, to include name and dosage of medication(s) and side effects	Requires FAA Decision
Chronic Tension or Cluster Headaches	All	Submit all pertinent medical records, current neurologic report, to include characteristics, frequency, severity, associated with neurologic phenomena, name and dosage of medication(s) and side effects	Requires FAA Decision
Migraines	All	Submit all pertinent medical records, current neurologic report, to include characteristics, frequency, severity, associated with neurologic phenomena, and name and dosage of medication(s) and side effects	**Initial Special Issuance** - Requires FAA Decision **Followup Special Issuance's** - See AASI Protocol

---

[5] Pain, in some conditions, may be acutely incapacitating. Chronic recurring headaches or pain syndromes often require medication for relief or prophylaxis, and, in most instances, the use of such medications are disqualifying because they may interfere with a pilot's alertness and functioning. The Examiner may issue a medical certificate to an applicant with a long-standing history of headaches if mild, seldom requiring more than simple analgesics, occur infrequently, are not incapacitating, and are not associated with neurological stigmata.

DISEASE/CONDITION	CLASS	EVALUATION DATA	DISPOSITION
Headaches			
Post-traumatic Headache	All	Submit all pertinent medical records, current neurologic report, name and dosage of medication(s) and side effects	Requires FAA Decision
DISEASE/CONDITION	**CLASS**	**EVALUATION DATA**	**DISPOSITION**
Hydrocephalus and Shunts			
Hydrocephalus, secondary to a known injury or disease process; or normal pressure	All	Submit all pertinent medical records, current neurologic report, to include name and dosage of medication(s) and side effects	Requires FAA Decision
Infections of the Nervous System			
Brain Abscess; Encephalitis; Meningitis; and Neurosyphilis	All	Complete neurological evaluation with appropriate laboratory and imaging studies	Requires FAA Decision

DISEASE/CONDITION	CLASS	EVALUATION DATA	DISPOSITION
Neurologic Conditions			
A disturbance of consciousness without satisfactory medical explanation of the cause	All	Submit all pertinent medical records, current neurologic report, to include name and dosage of medication(s) and side effects	Requires FAA Decision
Epilepsy[6] Rolandic Seizure *See below	All	Submit all pertinent medical records, current status report, to include name and dosage of medication(s) and side effects	Requires FAA Decision
Febrile Seizure[7] (Single episode)	All	Submit all pertinent medical records and a current status report	If occurred prior to age 5, without recurrence and off medications for 3 years - Issue Otherwise – Requires FAA Decision
Transient loss of nervous system function(s) without satisfactory medical explanation of the cause; e.g., transient global amnesia	All	Submit all pertinent medical records, current status report, to include name and dosage of medication(s) and side effects	Requires FAA Decision

---

[6] Unexplained syncope, single seizure. An applicant who has a history of epilepsy, a disturbance of consciousness without satisfactory medical explanation of the cause, or a transient loss of control of nervous system function(s) without satisfactory medical explanation of the cause must be denied or deferred by the Examiner. Rolandic seizures may be eligible for certification if the applicant is seizure free for 4 years and has a normal EEG. Consultation with the FAA required.

[7] Infrequently, the FAA has granted an Authorization under the special issuance section of part 67 (14 CFR 67.401) when a seizure disorder was present in childhood but the individual has been seizure-free for a number of years. Factors that would be considered in determining eligibility in such cases would be age at onset, nature and frequency of seizures, precipitating causes, and duration of stability without medication. Followup evaluations are usually necessary to confirm continued stability of an individual's condition if an Authorization is granted under the special issuance section of part 67 (14 CFR 67.401).

DISEASE/CONDITION	CLASS	EVALUATION DATA	DISPOSITION
Other Conditions			
Neurofibromatosis with Central Nervous System Involvement	All	Submit all pertinent medical information and current status medical report	Requires FAA Decision
Trigeminal Neuralgia	All	Submit all pertinent medical records, current neurologic report, name and dosage of medication(s) and side effects	Requires FAA Decision
Presence of any neurological condition or disease that potentially may incapacitate an individual			
Head Trauma associated with: Epidural or Subdural Hematoma; Focal Neurologic Deficit; Depressed Skull Fracture; or Unconsciousness or disorientation of more than 1 hour following injury	All	Submit all pertinent medical records, current status report, to include pre-hospital and emergency department records, operative reports, neurosurgical evaluation, name and dosage of medication(s) and side effects	Requires FAA Decision

DISEASE/CONDITION	CLASS	EVALUATION DATA	DISPOSITION
Spasticity, Weakness, or Paralysis of the Extremities			
Conditions that are stable and non-progressive may be considered for medical certification	All	Submit all pertinent medical records, current neurologic report, to include etiology, degree of involvement, period of stability, appropriate laboratory and imaging studies	Requires FAA Decision
Vertigo or Disequilibrium[8]			
Alternobaric Vertigo; Hyperventilation Syndrome; Meniere's Disease and Acute Peripheral Vestibulopathy; Nonfunctioning Labyrinths; or Orthostatic Hypotension	All	Submit all pertinent medical records, current neurologic report, name and dosage of medication(s) and side effects	Requires FAA Decision

---

[8] Numerous conditions may affect equilibrium, resulting in acute incapacitation or varying degrees of chronic recurring spatial disorientation. Prophylactic use of medications also may cause recurring spatial disorientation and affect pilot performance. In most instances, further neurological evaluation will be required to determine eligibility for medical certification.

ITEM 47. Psychiatric

CHECK EACH ITEM IN APPROPRIATE COLUMN	NORMAL	ABNORMAL
47. Psychiatric (Appearance, behavior, mood, communication, and memory)		

I. Code of Federal Regulations

All Classes: 14 CFR 67.107(a)(b)(c), 67.207(a)(b)(c), and 67.307(a)(b)(c)

(a) No established medical history or clinical diagnosis of any of the following:

(1) A personality disorder that is severe enough to have repeatedly manifested itself by overt acts.

(2) A psychosis. As used in this section, "psychosis" refers to a mental disorder in which:

(i) The individual has manifested delusions, hallucinations, grossly bizarre or disorganized behavior, or other commonly accepted symptoms of this condition; or

(ii) The individual may reasonably be expected to manifest delusions, hallucinations, grossly bizarre or disorganized behavior, or other commonly accepted symptoms of this condition.

(3) A bipolar disorder.

(4) Substance dependence, except where there is established clinical evidence, satisfactory to the Federal Air Surgeon, of recovery, including sustained total abstinence from the substance(s) for not less than the preceding 2 years. As used in this section -

(i) "Substance" includes: alcohol; other sedatives and hypnotics; anxiolytics; opioids; central nervous system stimulants such as cocaine, amphetamines, and similarly acting sympathomimetics; hallucinogens; phencyclidine or similarly acting arylcyclohexylamines; cannabis; inhalants; and other psychoactive drugs and chemicals; and

(ii) "Substance dependence" means a condition in which a person is dependent on a substance, other than tobacco or ordinary xanthine-containing (e.g., caffeine) beverages, as evidenced by-

(A) Increased tolerance
(B) Manifestation of withdrawal symptoms;
(C) Impaired control of use; or
(D) Continued use despite damage to physical health or impairment of

social, personal, or occupational functioning.

(b) No substance abuse within the preceding 2 years defined as:

   (1) Use of a substance in a situation in which that use was physically hazardous, if there has been at any other time an instance of the use of a substance also in a situation in which that use was physically hazardous;

   (2) A verified positive drug test result, an alcohol test result of 0.04 or greater alcohol concentration, or a refusal to submit to a drug or alcohol test required by the U.S. Department of Transportation or an agency of the U.S. Department of Transportation; or

   (3) Misuse of a substance that the Federal Air Surgeon, based on case history and appropriate, qualified medical judgment relating to the substance involved, finds-

      (i) Makes the person unable to safely perform the duties or exercise the privileges of the airman certificate applied for or held; or

      (ii) May reasonably be expected, for the maximum duration of the airman medical certificate applied for or held, to make the person unable to perform those duties or exercise those privileges.

(c) No other personality disorder, neurosis, or other mental condition that the Federal Air Surgeon, based on the case history and appropriate, qualified medical judgment relating to the condition involved, finds-

   (1) Makes the person unable to safely perform the duties or exercise the privileges of the airman certificate applied for or held; or

   (2) May reasonably be expected, for the maximum duration of the airman medical certificate applied for or held, to make the person unable to perform those duties or exercise those privileges.

(Also see **Items 18.m., 18.n.,** and **18.p.**)

II. Examination Techniques

The FAA does not expect the Examiner to perform a formal psychiatric examination. However, the Examiner should form a general impression of the emotional stability and mental state of the applicant. There is a need for discretion in the Examiner/applicant relationship consonant with the FAA's aviation safety mission and the concerns of all applicants regarding disclosure to a public agency of sensitive information that may not be pertinent to aviation safety. Examiners must be sensitive to this need while, at the same time, collect what is necessary for a certification decision. When a question arises, the Federal Air Surgeon encourages Examiners first to check this Guide for

Aviation Medical Examiners and other FAA informational documents. If the question remains unresolved, the Examiner should seek advice from a RFS or the Manager of the AMCD.

Review of the applicant's history as provided on the application form may alert the Examiner to gather further important factual information. Information about the applicant may be found in items related to age, pilot time, and class of certificate for which applied. Information about the present occupation and employer also may be helpful. If any psychotropic drugs are or have been used, followup questions are appropriate. Previous medical denials or aircraft accidents may be related to psychiatric problems.

Psychiatric information can be derived from the individual items in medical history (**Item 18**). Any affirmative answers to Item 18.m., " Mental disorders of any sort; depression, anxiety, etc.," or Item 18.p., "Suicide attempt," are significant. Any disclosure of current or previous alcohol or drug problems requires further clarification. A record of traffic violations may reflect certain personality problems or indicate an alcohol problem. Affirmative answers related to rejection by military service or a military medical discharge require elaboration. Reporting symptoms such as headaches or dizziness, or even heart or stomach trouble, may reflect a history of anxiety rather than a primary medical problem in these areas. Sometimes, the information applicants give about their previous diagnoses is incorrect, either because the applicant is unsure of the correct information or because the applicant chooses to minimize past difficulties. If there was a hospital admission for any emotionally related problem, it will be necessary to obtain the entire record.

Valuable information can be derived from the casual conversation that occurs during the physical examination. Some of this conversation will reveal information about the family, the job, and special interests. Even some personal troubles may be revealed at this time. The Examiner's questions should not be stilted or follow a regular pattern; instead, they should be a natural extension of the Examiner's curiosity about the person being examined. Information about the motivation for medical certification and interest in flying may be revealing. A formal Mental Status Examination is unnecessary. For example, it is not necessary to ask about time, place, or person to discover whether the applicant is oriented. Information about the flow of associations, mood, and memory, is generally available from the usual interactions during the examination. Indication of cognitive problems may become apparent during the examination. Such problems with concentration, attention, or confusion during the examination or slower, vague responses should be noted and may be cause for deferral.

The Examiner should make observations about the following specific elements and should note on the form any gross or notable deviations from normal:

1. Appearance (abnormal if dirty, disheveled, odoriferous, or unkempt);

2. Behavior (abnormal if uncooperative, bizarre, or inexplicable);

3. Mood (abnormal if excessively angry, sad, euphoric, or labile);

4. Communication (abnormal if incomprehensible, does not answer questions directly);

5. Memory (abnormal if unable to recall recent events); and

6. Cognition (abnormal if unable to engage in abstract thought, or if delusional or hallucinating).

Significant observations during this part of the medical examination should be recorded in Item 60, of the application form. The Examiner, upon identifying any significant problems, should defer issuance of the medical certificate and report findings to the FAA. This could be accomplished by contacting a RFS or the Manager of the AMCD.

III. Aerospace Medical Disposition

A. General Considerations. It must be pointed out that considerations for safety, which in the "mental" area are related to a compromise of judgment and emotional control or to diminished mental capacity with loss of behavioral control, are not the same as concerns for emotional health in everyday life. Some problems may have only a slight impact on an individual's overall capacities and the quality of life but may nevertheless have a great impact on safety. Conversely, many emotional problems that are of therapeutic and clinical concern have no impact on safety.

B. Denials. The FAA has concluded that certain psychiatric conditions are such that their presence or a past history of their presence is sufficient to suggest a significant potential threat to aviation safety. It is, therefore, incumbent upon the Examiner to be aware of any indications of these conditions currently or in the past, and to deny or defer issuance of the medical certificate to an applicant who has a history of these conditions. An applicant who has a current diagnosis or history of these conditions may request the FAA to grant an Authorization under the special issuance section of part 67 (14 CFR 67.401) and, based upon individual considerations, the FAA may grant such an issuance.

All applicants with any of the following conditions must be denied or deferred:

Attention Deficit Disorder   Substance Abuse
Bipolar Disorder   Substance Dependence
Personality Disorder   Suicide Attempt
Psychosis

In some instances, the following conditions may also warrant denial or deferral:

Adjustment Disorder
Bereavement; Dysthmic; or Minor Depression
Use of Psychotropic Medications for Smoking Cessation

NOTE: The use of a psychotropic drug is disqualifying for aeromedical certification purposes. This includes all sedatives, tranquilizers, antipsychotic drugs, antidepressant drugs (including SSRI's -see exceptions below), analeptics, anxiolytics, and hallucinogens. The Examiner should defer issuance and forward the medical records to the AMCD.

C. Use of Antidepressant Medications. The FAA has determined that airmen requesting first, second, or third class medical certificates while being treated with one of four specific selective serotonin reuptake inhibitors (SSRIs) may be considered. The Authorization decision is made on a case by case basis. **The Examiner may not issue.**

If the applicant opts to discontinue use of the SSRI, the Examiner must notate in Block 60, Comments on History and Findings, on FAA Form 8500-8 and defer issuance. To reapply for regular issuance, the applicant must be off the SSRI for a minimum of 60 days with a favorable report from the treating physician indicating stable mood and no aeromedically significant side effects. See SSRI Decision Path I

An applicant may be considered for an FAA Authorization of a Special Issuance (SI) of a Medical Certificate (Authorization) if:

1.) The applicant has one of the following diagnoses:
- Major depressive disorder (mild to moderate) either single episode or recurrent episode
- Dysthymic disorder
- Adjustment disorder with depressed mood
- Any non-depression related condition for which the SSRI is used

2.) For a minimum of 12 continuous months prior, the applicant has been clinically stable as well as on a stable dose of medication without any aeromedically significant side effects and/or an increase in symptoms. If the applicant has been on the medication under 12 months, the Examiner must advise that 12 months of continuous use is required before SI consideration.

3.) The SSRI used is one the following (single use only):
- Fluoxetine (Prozac)
- Sertraline (Zoloft)
- Citalopram (Celexa)
- Escialopram (Lexapro)

If the applicant is on a SSRI that is not listed above, the Examiner must advise that the medication is not acceptable for SI consideration.

4.) The applicant DOES NOT have symptoms or history of:
- Psychosis
- Suicidal ideation
- Electro convulsive therapy
- Treatment with multiple SSRIs concurrently

- Multi-agent drug protocol use (prior use of other psychiatric drugs in conjunction with SSRIs.)

If applicant meets the all of the above criteria and wishes to continue use of the SSRI, advise the applicant that he/she must be further evaluated by a Human Intervention Motivation Study (HIMS) AME. See SSRI Decision Path II (HIMS AME). The HIMS AME will also conduct the follow up evaluation after initial issuance. See SSRI Follow Up Path.

For more policy information, see Federal Register/ Vol. 75, No 64/ Monday, April 5, 2010/ Rules and Regulations at http://edocket.access.gpo.gov/2010/pdf/2010-7527.pdf

SSRI Decision Path - I

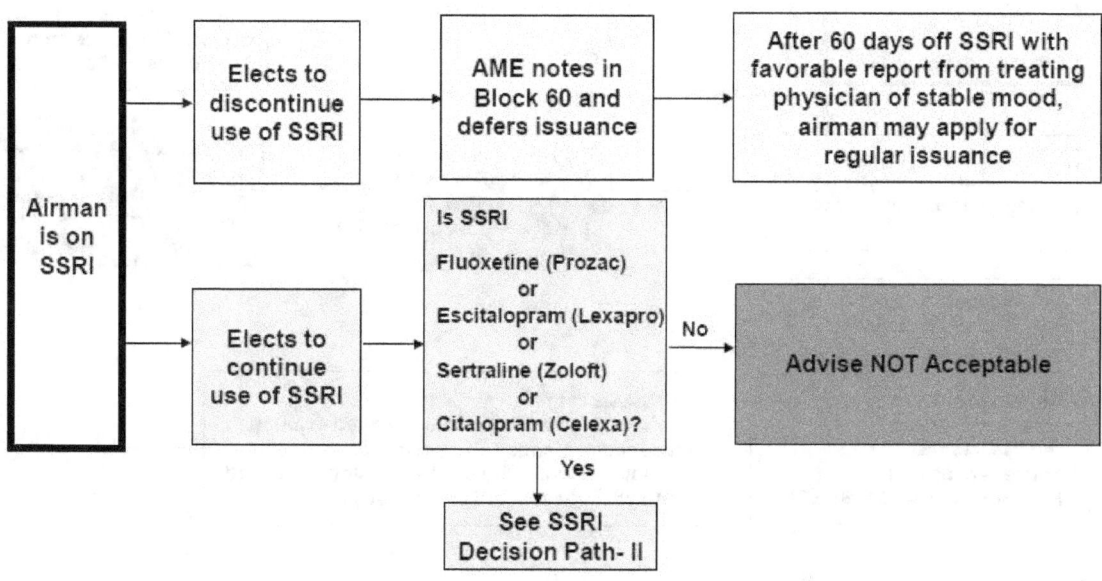

SSRI Decision Path – II (HIMS AME)

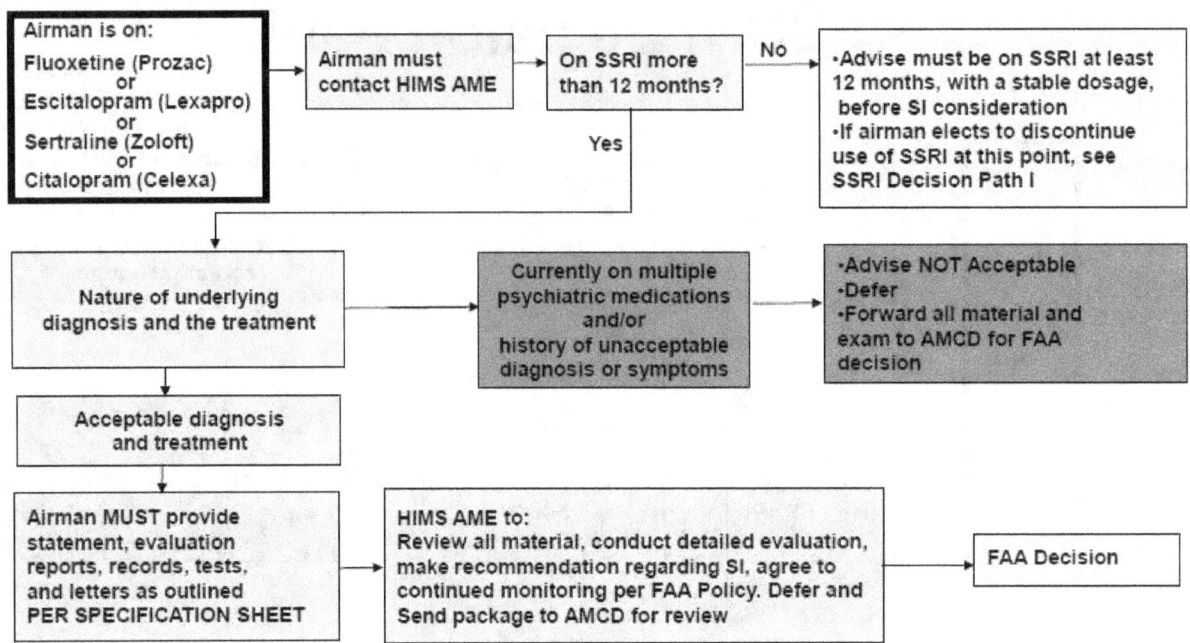

SSRI Follow Up Path

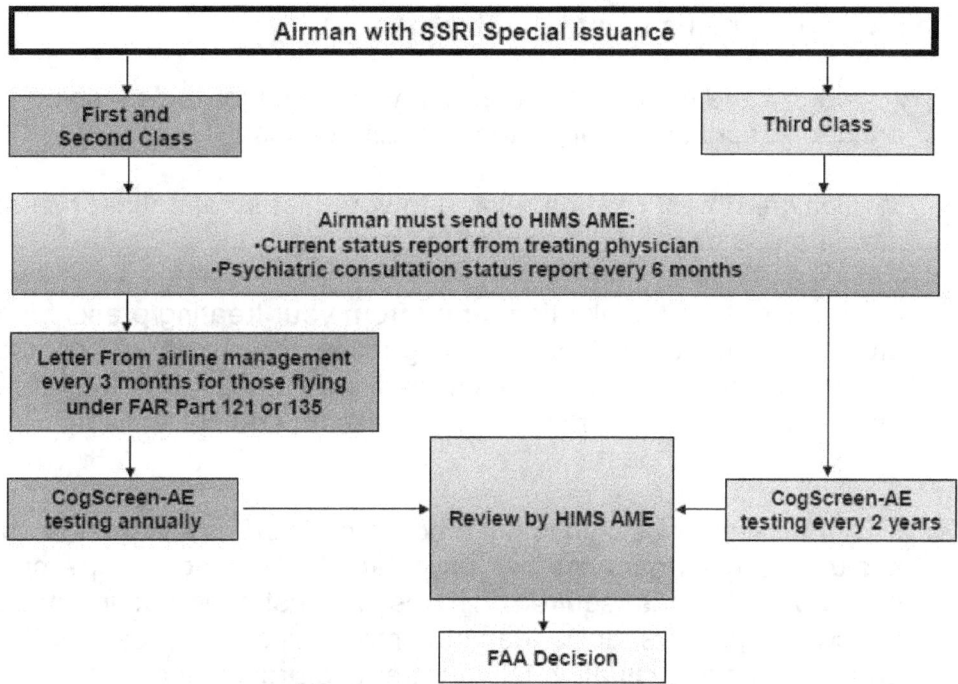

'Note: HIMS AME may issue if subsequent certification exam does not coincide with required neurocognitive testing and if all follow-up material is acceptable.
When CogScreen is due, send records to Medical Appeals, AAM-240, Washington, DC.

SSRI SPECIFICATION SHEET

The following items must be submitted:

1. A written statement from you and in your own words describing your history of antidepressant usage and mental health status.

2. Medical/treatment records related to your history of antidepressant usage from the date you began treatment to the present.

3. A current detailed evaluation report from your treating/prescribing physician attesting to and describing your diagnoses, the length and course of treatment, the dosage of the antidepressant medication taken, and the presence of any side effects experienced from the antidepressant you currently take and/or that you have taken in the past.

4. If your treating physician is not a board certified psychiatrist, a current detailed evaluation by a board certified psychiatrist regarding your psychiatric and behavioral status is required. The psychiatrist must document that he/she has reviewed your personal written statement, all of your treatment/medical records, and the current evaluation by your treating/prescribing physician.

5. A neuropsychologist's report with the report of the results of a **CogScreen - Aeromedical Edition (AE)** neurocognitive psychological test including a copy of the test computer score reports.

6. If you have held a first- or second-class airman medical certificate and have flown for a commercial carrier within the last 2 years, obtain a letter from airline management (Chief Pilot or designee) attesting to your competence, crew interaction and mood (if available).

7. A detailed evaluation by your HIMS AME. The evaluation must address the following:

   - A statement verifying he/she has reviewed the above documents.
   - A current psychiatric status of the applicant.
   - A comment regarding a recommendation for a Special Issuance medical certificate.
   - The HIMS AME must include a statement agreeing to serve as your independent medical sponsor.

The following is a table that lists the most common conditions of aeromedical significance, and course of action that should be taken by the examiner as defined by the protocol and disposition in the table. Medical certificates must not be issued to an applicant with medical conditions that require deferral, or for any condition not listed in the table that may result in sudden or subtle incapacitation without consulting the AMCD or the RFS. Medical documentation must be submitted for any condition in order to support an issuance of an airman medical certificate.

DISEASE/CONDITION	CLASS	EVALUATION DATA	DISPOSTION
Psychiatric Conditions			
Adjustment Disorders	All	Submit all pertinent medical information and clinical status report	If stable, resolved, no associated disturbance of thought, no recurrent episodes, and psychotropic medication(s) used for less than 6 months and discontinued for at least 3 months - Issue Otherwise - Requires FAA Decision
Attention Deficit Disorder	All	Submit all pertinent medical information and clinical status report to include documenting the period of use, name and dosage of any medication(s), and side-effects. If submitting neurocognitive test data, the applicant must have a drug screen for ADD medications done within 24 hours of the neurocognitive testing and submit the results.	Requires FAA Decision

DISEASE/CONDITION	CLASS	EVALUATION DATA	DISPOSTION
Psychiatric Conditions			
Bipolar Disorder	All	See 3. below	Requires FAA Decision
Bereavement; Dysthmic; or Minor Depression	All	Submit all pertinent medical information and clinical status report	If stable, resolved, no associated disturbance of thought, no recurrent episodes, and; a). psychotropic medication(s) used for less than 6 months and discontinued for at least 3 months – Issue b). No use of psychotropic medication(s) - Issue Otherwise - Requires FAA Decision
Depression requiring the use of antidepressant medications	All	Submit all pertinent medical information and clinical status report See Use of Antidepressant Medication Policy	Requires FAA Decision
Personality Disorders	All	See 1. below	Requires FAA Decision
Psychosis	All	See 2. below	Requires FAA Decision
Pyschotropic medications for Smoking Cessation	All	Document period of use, name and dosage of medication(s) and side-effects	If medication(s) discontinued for at least 30 days and w/o side-effects - Issue Otherwise – Requires FAA Decision
Substance Abuse	All	See 6. below	Requires FAA Decision
Substance Dependence	All	See 5. below	Requires FAA Decision
Suicide Attempt	All	Submit all pertinent medical information required	Requires FAA Decision

1. The category of personality disorders severe enough to have repeatedly manifested itself by overt acts refers to diagnosed personality disorders that involve what is called "acting out" behavior. These personality problems relate to poor social judgment, impulsivity, and disregard or antagonism toward authority, especially rules and regulations. A history of long-standing behavioral problems, whether major (criminal) or relatively minor (truancy, military misbehavior, petty criminal and civil indiscretions, and social instability), usually occurs with these disorders. Driving infractions and previous failures to follow aviation regulations are critical examples of these acts.

   Certain personality disorders and other mental disorders that include conditions of limited duration and/or widely varying severity may be disqualifying. Under this category, the FAA is especially concerned with significant depressive episodes requiring treatment, even outpatient therapy. If these episodes have been severe enough to cause some disruption of vocational or educational activity, or if they have required medication or involved suicidal ideation, the application should be deferred or denied issuance.

   Some personality disorders and situational dysphorias may be considered disqualifying for a limited time. These include such conditions as gross immaturity and some personality disorders not involving or manifested by overt acts.

2. Psychotic Disorders are characterized by a loss of reality testing in the form of delusions, hallucinations, or disorganized thoughts. They may be chronic, intermittent, or occur in a single episode. They may also occur as accompanying symptoms in other psychiatric conditions including but not limited to bipolar disorder (e.g. bipolar disorder with psychotic features), major depression (e.g. major depression with psychotic features), borderline personality disorder, etc. **All applicants with such a diagnosis must be denied or deferred.**

3. Bipolar Disorders are considered on a continuum as part of a spectrum of disorders where there are significant alternations in mood. Generally, only one episode of manic or hypomanic behavior is necessary to make the diagnosis. Please note that cyclothymic disorder is part of this spectrum. Even if the bipolar disorder does not have accompanying symptoms that reach the level of psychosis, the disorder can be so disruptive of judgment and functioning (especially mania) as to pose a significant risk to aviation safety. Impaired judgment does occur even in the milder form of the disease. **All applicants with a diagnosis of Bipolar Disorder must be denied or deferred.**

4. Although they may be rare in occurrence, severe anxiety problems, especially anxiety and phobias associated with some aspect of flying, are considered significant. Organic mental disorders that cause a cognitive defect, even if the applicant is not psychotic, are considered disqualifying whether they are due to

trauma, toxic exposure, or arteriosclerotic or other degenerative changes. (See **Item 18.m.**).

5. Substance dependence refers to the use of substances of dependence, which include alcohol and other drugs (i.e., PCP, sedatives and hypnotics, anxiolytics, marijuana, cocaine, opioids, amphetamines, hallucinogens, and other psychoactive drugs or chemicals). Substance dependence is defined and specified as a disqualifying medical condition. It is disqualifying unless there is clinical evidence, satisfactory to the Federal Air Surgeon, of recovery, including sustained total abstinence from the substance for not less than the preceding 2 years.

   Substance dependence is evidenced by one or more of the following: increased tolerance, manifestation of withdrawal symptoms, impaired control of use, or continued use despite damage to physical health or impairment of social, personal, or occupational functioning. Substance dependence is accompanied by various deleterious effects on physical health as well as personal or social functioning. There are many other indicators of substance dependence in the history and physical examination. Treatment for substance dependence-related problems, arrests, including charges of driving under the influence of drugs or alcohol, and vocational or marital disruption related to drugs or alcohol consumption are important indicators. Alcohol on the breath at the time of a routine physical examination should arouse a high index of suspicion. Consumption of drugs or alcohol sufficient to cause liver damage is an indication of the presence of alcoholism.

6. Substance abuse includes the use of the above substances under any one of the following conditions:

   a. Use of a substance in the last 2 years in which the use was physically hazardous (e.g., DUI or DWI) if there has been at any other time an instance of the use of a substance also in a situation in which the use was physically hazardous;

   b. If a person has received a verified positive drug test result under an anti-drug program of the Department of Transportation or one of its administrations; or

   c. The Federal Air Surgeon finds that an applicant's misuse of a substance makes him or her unable to safely perform the duties or exercise the privileges of the airman certificate applied for or held, or that may reasonably be expected, for the maximum duration of the airman medical certificate applied for or held, to make the applicant unable to perform those duties or exercise those privileges.

   Substance dependence and substance abuse are specified as disqualifying medical conditions.

ITEM 48. General Systemic

CHECK EACH ITEM IN APPROPRIATE COLUMN	NORMAL	ABNORMAL
48. General Systemic		

I. Code of Federal Regulations

All Classes: 14 CFR 67.113(a)(b)(c), 67.213(a)(b)(c), and 67.313(a)(b)(c)

(a) No established medical history or clinical diagnosis of diabetes mellitus that requires insulin or any other hypoglycemic drug for control.

(b) No other organic, functional, or structural disease, defect, or limitation that the Federal Air Surgeon, based on the case history and appropriate, qualified medical judgment relating to the condition involved, finds -

    (1) Makes the person unable to safely perform the duties or exercise the privileges of the airman certificate applied for or held; or

    (2) May reasonably be expected, for the maximum duration of the airman medical certificate applied for or held, to make the person unable to perform those duties or exercise those privileges.

(c) No medication or other treatment that the Federal Air Surgeon, based on the case history and appropriate, qualified medical judgment relating to the medication or other treatment involved, finds -

    (1) Makes the person unable to safely perform the duties or exercise the privileges of the airman certificate applied for or held; or

    (2) May reasonably be expected, for the maximum duration of the airman medical certificate applied for or held, to make the person unable to perform those duties or exercise those privileges.

II. Examination Techniques

A protocol for examinations applicable to Item 48 is not provided because the necessary history-taking, observation, and other examination techniques used in examining other systems have already revealed much of what can be known about the status of the applicant's endocrine and other systems. For example, the examination of the skin alone can reveal important signs of thyroid dysfunction, Addison's disease, Cushing's disease, and several other endocrine disorders. The eye may reflect a thyroid disorder (exophthalmos) or diabetes (retinopathy).

When the Examiner reaches Item 48 in the course of the examination of an applicant, it is recommended that the Examiner take a moment to review and determine if key procedures have been performed in conjunction with examinations made under other items, and to determine the relevance of any positive or abnormal findings.

III. Aerospace Medical Disposition

The following is a table that lists the most common conditions of aeromedical significance, and course of action that should be taken by the examiner as defined by the protocol and disposition in the table. Medical certificates must not be issued to an applicant with medical conditions that require deferral, or for any condition not listed in the table that may result in sudden or subtle incapacitation without consulting the AMCD or the RFS. Medical documentation must be submitted for any condition in order to support an issuance of an airman medical certificate.

DISEASE/CONDITION	CLASS	EVALUATION DATA	DISPOSITION
Blood and Blood-Forming Tissue Disease			
Anemia	All	Submit a current status report and all pertinent medical reports. Include a CBC, and any other tests deemed necessary	Requires FAA Decision
Hemophilia	All	Submit a current status report and all pertinent medical reports. Include frequency, severity and location of bleeding sites	Requires FAA Decision
Other disease of the blood or blood-forming tissues that could adversely affect performance of airman duties	All	Submit a current status report and all pertinent medical reports	Requires FAA Decision
Polycythemia	All	Submit a current status report and all pertinent medical reports; include CBC	Requires FAA Decision

DISEASE/CONDITION	CLASS	EVALUATION DATA	DISPOSITION
Diabetes, Metabolic Syndrome, and/or Insulin Resistance			
Diabetes Insipidus	All	Submit all pertinent medical records; current status to include names and dosage of medication(s) and side effects	Requires FAA Decision
Diet Controlled Diabetes Mellitus and Metabolic Syndrome,	All	See Diet Controlled Diabetes Mellitus and Metabolic Syndrome Protocol	If no glycosuria and normal Hgba1c - Issue
Insulin Treated Diabetes Mellitus I & II	1st & 2nd	Not currently granting Special Issuance	Requires FAA Decision
	3rd	See Insulin Treated Diabetes Mellitus I & II Protocol	Requires FAA Decision
Medication Controlled (non insulin) Diabetes Mellitus II	All	See Medication Controlled (non insulin) Diabetes Mellitus II Protocol	**Initial Special Issuance** - Requires FAA Decision **Followup Special Issuance's** - See AASI Protocol
Medication Controlled Metabolic Syndrome (Glucose Intolerance, Impaired Glucose tolerance, Impaired Fasting Glucose, Insulin Resistance, and Pre-Diabetes)	All	See Medication Controlled Metabolic Syndrome Protocol	**Initial Special Issuance** – Requires FAA Decision

DISEASE/CONDITION	CLASS	EVALUATION DATA	DISPOSITION
Endocrine Disorders			
Acromegaly	All	Submit all pertinent medical records; current status to include names and dosage of medication(s) and side effects	Requires FAA Decision
Addison's Disease	All	Submit all pertinent medical records; current status to include names and dosage of medication(s) and side effects	Requires FAA Decision
Cushing's Disease or Syndrome	All	Submit all pertinent medical records; current status to include names and dosage of medication(s) and side effects	Requires FAA Decision
Hypoglycemia, whether functional or a result of pancreatic tumor	All	Submit all pertinent medical records; current status to include names and dosage of medication(s) and side effects	Requires FAA Decision
Hyperparathyroidism	All	Submit all pertinent medical records; current status;include names and dosage of medication(s) and side effects, and current serum calcium and phosphorus levels	If status post-surgery, disease controlled, stable and no sequela - Issue Otherwise - Requires FAA Decision
Hypoparathyroidism	All	Submit all pertinent medical records; current status; include names and dosage of medication(s) and side effects and current serum calcium and phosphorus levels	Requires FAA Decision

DISEASE/CONDITION	CLASS	EVALUATION DATA	DISPOSITION
Endocrine Disorders			
Hyperthyroidism	All	Submit all pertinent medical records; current status to include names and dosage of medication(s) and side effects and current TFTs	**Initial Special Issuance** – Requires FAA Decision **Followup Special Issuances** – See AASI Protocol
Hypothyroidism	All	Submit all pertinent medical records; current status to include names and dosage of medication(s) and side effects and current TFTs	**Initial Special Issuance** – Requires FAA Decision (Call FAA for verbal clearance if airman presents current lab reports) **Followup Special Issuances** – See AASI Protocol
Proteinuria & Glycosuria	All	Submit all pertinent medical records; current status to include names and dosage of medication(s) and side effects	Trace or 1+ protein and glucose intolerance ruled out - Issue Otherwise - Requires FAA Decision
Human Immunodeficiency Virus (HIV)			
Acquired Immunodeficiency Syndrome (AIDS)	All	See HIV Protocol	Requires FAA Decision
Human Immunodeficiency Virus (HIV)	All	See HIV Protocol	Requires FAA Decision

DISEASE/CONDITION	CLASS	EVALUATION DATA	DISPOSITION
Neoplasms			
Breast Cancer	All	Submit all pertinent medical records, operative/ pathology reports, current oncological status report, including tumor markers, and any other testing; include duration of symptoms, name and dosage of drugs and side effects	**Initial Special Issuance** - Requires FAA Decision **Followup Special Issuance's** - See AASI Protocol
Also see: Acoustic Neuroma Colon/ Rectal Cancer and other Abdominal Malignancies G-U System Cancers Kaposi's Sarcoma Leukemias and Lymphomas Malignant Melanomas Eye Tumors			

ITEM 49. Hearing

49. Hearing	Record Audiometric Speech Discrimination Score Below
Conversational Voice Test at 6 Feet ☐ Pass ☐ Fail	

I. Code of Federal Regulations

All Classes: 14 CFR 67.105(a)(b)(c), 67.205(a)(b)(c), and 67.305(a)(b)(c)

(a) The person shall demonstrate acceptable hearing by at least one of the following tests:

  (1) Demonstrate an ability to hear an average conversational voice in a quiet room, using both ears, at a distance of 6 feet from the examiner, with the back turned to the examiner.

  (2) Demonstrate an acceptable understanding of speech as determined by audiometric speech discrimination testing to a score of at least 70 percent obtained in one ear or in a sound field environment.

  (3) Provide acceptable results of pure tone audiometric testing of unaided hearing acuity according to the following table of worst acceptable thresholds, using the calibration standards of the American National Standards Institute, 1969 (11 West 42nd Street, New York, NY 10036):

Frequency (Hz)	500 Hz	1000 Hz	2000 Hz	3000 Hz
Better ear (Db)	35	30	30	40
Poorer ear (Db)	35	50	50	60

(b) No disease or condition of the middle or internal ear, nose, oral cavity, pharynx, or larynx that-

  (1) Interferes with, or is aggravated by, flying or may reasonably be expected to do so; or

  (2) Interferes with, or may reasonably be expected to interfere with, clear and effective speech communication.

(c) No disease or condition manifested by, or that may reasonably be expected to be manifested by, vertigo or a disturbance of equilibrium.

II. Examination Equipment and Techniques

A. Order of Examinations

1. The applicant must demonstrate an ability to hear an average conversational voice in a quiet room, using both ears, at a distance of 6 feet from the Examiner, with the back turned to the Examiner.

2. If an applicant fails the conversational voice test, the Examiner may administer pure tone audiometric testing of unaided hearing acuity according to the following table of worst acceptable thresholds, using the calibration standards of the American National Standards Institute, 1969:

Frequency (Hz)	500 Hz	1000 Hz	2000 Hz	3000 Hz
Better ear (Db)	35	30	30	40
Poorer ear (Db)	35	50	50	60

If the applicant fails an audiometric test and the conversational voice test had not been administered, the conversational voice test should be performed to determine if the standard applicable to that test can be met.

3. If an applicant is unable to pass either the conversational voice test or the pure tone audiometric test, then an audiometric speech discrimination test should be administered. A passing score is at least 70 percent obtained in one ear at an intensity of no greater than 65 Db.

B. Discussion

1. Conversational voice test. For all classes of certification, the applicant must demonstrate hearing of an average conversational voice in a quiet room, using both ears, at 6 feet, with the back turned to the Examiner. The Examiner should not use only sibilants (S-sounding test materials). If the applicant is able to repeat correctly the test numbers or words, "pass" should be noted and recorded on FAA Form 8500-8, Item 49. If the applicant is unable to hear a normal conversational voice then "fail" should be marked and one of the following tests may be administered.

2. Standard. For all classes of certification, the applicant may be examined by pure tone audiometry as an alternative to conversational voice testing or upon failing the conversational voice test. If the applicant fails the pure tone audiometric test and has not been tested by conversational voice, that test may be administered. The requirements expressed as audiometric standards according to a table of acceptable thresholds (American National Standards Institute [ANSI], 1969, calibration) are as follows:

EAR(All classes of medical certification)				
Frequency (Hz)	500 Hz	1000 Hz	2000 Hz	3000 Hz
Better ear (Db)	35	30	30	40
Poorer ear (Db)	35	50	50	60

3. Audiometric Speech Discrimination. Upon failing both conversational voice and pure tone audiometric test, an audiometric speech discrimination test should be administered (usually by an otologist or audiologist). The applicant must score at least 70 percent at intensity no greater than 65 Db in either ear.

C. Equipment

1. Approval. The FAA does not approve or designate specific audiometric equipment for use in medical certification. Equipment used for FAA testing must accurately and reliably cover the required frequencies and have adequate threshold step features. Because every audiometer manufactured in the United States for
screening and diagnostic purposes is built to meet appropriate standards, most audiometers should be acceptable *if they are maintained in proper calibration* and are used in an adequately quiet place.

2. Calibration. It is critical that any audiometer be periodically calibrated to ensure its continued accuracy. Annual calibration is recommended. Also recommended is the further safeguard of obtaining an occasional audiogram on a "known" subject or staff member between calibrations, especially at any time that a test result unexpectedly varies significantly from the hearing levels clinically expected. This testing provides an approximate "at threshold" calibration. The Examiner should ensure that the audiometer is calibrated to ANSI standards or if calibrated to the older ASA/USASI standards, the appropriate correction is applied (see paragraph 3 below).

3. ASA/ANSI. Older audiometers were often calibrated to meet the standards specified by the USA Standards Institute (USASI), formerly the American Standards Association (ASA). These standards were based upon a U.S. Public Health Service survey. Newer audiometers are calibrated so that the zero hearing threshold level is now based on laboratory measurements rather than on the survey. In 1969, the American National Standards Institute (ANSI) incorporated these new measurements. Audiometers built to this standard have instruments or dials that read in ANSI values. For these reasons, *it is very important that every audiogram submitted (for values reported in Item 49 on FAA Form 8500-8) include a note indicating whether it is ASA or ANSI.* Only then can the FAA standards be appropriately applied. ASA or USASI values can be converted to ANSI by adding corrections as follows:

Frequency (Hz)	500 Hz	1,000 Hz	2,000 Hz	3,000 Hz
Decibels Added*	14	10	8.5	8.5

* The decibels added figure is the amount added to ASA or USASI at each specific frequency to convert to ANSI or older equivalent ISO values.

III. Aerospace Medical Disposition

1. Special Issuance of Medical Certificates. Applicants who do not meet the auditory standards may be found eligible for a SODA. An applicant seeking a SODA must make the request in writing to the Aerospace Medicine Certification Division, AAM-300. A determination of qualifications will be made on the basis of a special medical examination by an ENT consultant, a MFT, or operational experience.

2. Bilateral Deafness. If otherwise qualified, the AMCD may issue a combination medical/student pilot certificate with the limitation VALID FOR STUDENT PILOT PURPOSES ONLY as well as the limitation NOT VALID FOR CONTROL ZONES OR AREAS WHERE RADIO COMMUNICATION IS REQUIRED. This will enable the applicant to proceed with training to the point of a private pilot checkride. See **Items 25-30.**

   When the student pilot's instructor confirms the student's eligibility for a private pilot checkride, the applicant should submit a written request to the AMCD, for an authorization for a MFT. This test will be given by an FAA inspector in conjunction with the checkride. If the applicant successfully completes the test, the FAA will issue a third-class medical certificate and SODA. Pilot activities will be restricted to areas in which radio communication is not required.

3. Hearing Aids. If the applicant requires the use of hearing aids to meet the standard, issue the certificate with the following restriction:

   VALID ONLY WITH USE OF HEARING AMPLIFICATION

   Some pilots who normally wear hearing aids to assist in communicating while on the ground report that they elect not to wear them while flying. They prefer to use the volume amplification of the radio headphone. Some use the headphone on one ear for radio communication and the hearing aid in the other for cockpit communications.

ITEMS 50- 54. Ophthalmologic Disorder

ITEM 50. Distant Vision

50. Distant Vision		
Right	20/	Corrected to 20/
Left	20/	Corrected to 20/
Both	20/	Corrected to 20/

I. Code of Federal Regulations

First- and Second-Classes: 14 CFR 67.103(a) and 67.203(a)

(a) Distant visual acuity of 20/20 or better in each eye separately, with or without corrective lenses. If corrective lenses (spectacles or contact lenses) are necessary for 20/20 vision, the person may be eligible only on the condition that corrective lenses are worn while exercising the privileges of an airman certificate

Third-Class: 14 CFR 67.303(a)

(a) Distant visual acuity of 20/40 or better in each eye separately, with or without corrective lenses. If corrective lenses (spectacles or contact lenses) are necessary for 20/40 vision, the person may be eligible only on the condition that corrective lenses are worn while exercising the privileges of an airman certificate.

II. Examination Equipment and Techniques

Equipment:

1. Snellen 20-foot eye chart may be used as follows:

    a. The Snellen chart should be illuminated by a 100-watt incandescent lamp placed 4 feet in front of and slightly above the chart.

    b. The chart or screen should be placed 20 feet from the applicant's eyes and the 20/20 line should be placed 5 feet 4 inches above the floor.

    c. A metal, opaque plastic, or cardboard occluder should be used to cover the eye not being examined.

    d. The examining room should be darkened with the exception of the illuminated chart or screen.

    e. If the applicant wears corrective lenses, the uncorrected acuity should be determined first, then corrected acuity. If the applicant wears contact lenses, see the recommendations in Chapter 3. Items 31-34, Section II, #5,

    f. Common errors:

        1. Failure to shield the applicant's eyes from extraneous light.

        2. Permitting the applicant to view the chart with both eyes.

        3. Failure to observe the applicant's face to detect squinting.

        4. Incorrect sizing of projected chart letters for a 20-foot distance.

5. Failure to focus the projector sharply.

6. Failure to obtain the corrected acuity when the applicant wears glasses.

7. Failure to note and to require the removal of contact lenses.

2. Acceptable Substitutes for Distant Vision Testing: any commercial available visual acuities and heterphoria testing devices.

   There are specific approved substitute testers for color vision, which may not include some commercially available vision testing machines. For an approved list, see Item 52. Color Vision.

3. Directions furnished by the manufacturer or distributor should be followed when using the acceptable substitute devices for the above testing.

Examination Techniques:

1. Each eye will be tested separately, and both eyes together.

III. Aerospace Medical Disposition

A. When corrective lenses are required to meet the standards, an appropriate limitation will be placed on the medical certificate. For example, when lenses are needed for distant vision only:

HOLDER SHALL WEAR CORRECTIVE LENSES

For multiple vision defects involving distant and/or intermediate and/or near vision when one set of monofocal lenses corrects for all, the limitation is:

HOLDER SHALL WEAR CORRECTIVE LENSES

For combined defective distant and near visual acuity where multifocal lenses are required, the appropriate limitation is:

HOLDER SHALL WEAR LENSES THAT CORRECT FOR DISTANT VISION AND POSSESS GLASSES THAT CORRECT FOR NEAR VISION

For multiple vision defects involving distant, near, and intermediate visual acuity when more than one set of lenses is required to correct for all vision defects, the appropriate limitation is:

HOLDER SHALL WEAR LENSES THAT CORRECT FOR DISTANT VISION AND POSSESS GLASSES THAT CORRECT FOR NEAR AND INTERMEDIATE VISION

B. An applicant who fails to meet vision standards and has no SODA that covers the extent of the visual acuity defect found on examination may obtain further FAA consideration for grant of an Authorization under the special issuance section of part 67 (14 CFR 67.401) for medical certification by submitting a report of an eye evaluation. The Examiner can help to expedite the review procedure by forwarding a copy of FAA Form 8500-7, Report of Eye Evaluation, that has been completed by an eye specialist (optometrist or ophthmologist) [1].

C. Applicants who do not meet the visual standards should be referred to a specialist for evaluation. Applicants with visual acuity or ocular muscle balance problems may be referred to an eye specialist of the applicant's choice. The FAA Form 8500-7, Report of Eye Evaluation, should be provided to the specialist by the Examiner.

Any applicant eligible for a medical certificate through special issuance under these guidelines shall pass a MFT, which may be arranged through the appropriate agency medical authority. While waiting to complete a MFT, an applicant who is otherwise qualified for certification may be issued a medical certificate, which must contain the limitation "Valid for Student Pilot Privileges Only."

D. Amblyopia. In amblyopia ex anopsia, the visual acuity of one eye is decreased without presence of organic eye disease, usually because of strabismus or anisometropia in childhood. In amblyopia ex anopsia, the visual acuity loss is simply recorded in Item 50 of FAA form 8500-8, and visual standards are applied as usual. If the standards are not met, a report of eye evaluation, FAA Form 8500-7, should be submitted for consideration.

---

[1] In obtaining special eye evaluations in respect to the airman medical certification program or the air traffic controller health program, reports from an eye specialist are acceptable when the condition being evaluated relates to a determination of visual acuity, refractive error, or mechanical function of the eye. The FAA Form 8500-7, Report of Eye Evaluation, is a form that is designed for use by either optometrists or ophthalmologists.

ITEM 51.a. Near Vision

51.a. Near Vision		
Right	20/	Corrected to 20/
Left	20/	Corrected to 20/
Both	20/	Corrected to 20/

ITEM 51.b. Intermediate Vision

51.b. Intermediate Vision – 32 Inches		
Right	20/	Corrected to 20/
Left	20/	Corrected to 20/
Both	20/	Corrected to 20/

I. Code of Federal Regulations

First- and Second-Classes: 14 CFR 67.103(b) and 67.203(b)

(b) Near vision of 20/40 or better, Snellen equivalent, at 16 inches in each eye separately, with or without corrective lenses. If age 50 or older, near vision of 20/40 or better, Snellen equivalent, at both 16 inches and 32 inches in each eye separately, with or without corrective lenses.

Third-Class: 14 CFR 67.303(b)

(b) Near vision of 20/40 or better, Snellen equivalent, at 16 inches in each eye separately, with or without corrective lenses.

II. Equipment and Examination Techniques

Equipment:

1. FAA Form 8500-1, Near Vision Acuity Test Chart, dated April 1993.

2. For testing near at 16 inches and intermediate at 32 inches, acceptable substitutes: any commercially available visual acuities and heterophoria testing devices. For testing of intermediate vision, some equipment may require additional apparatus.

There are specific approved substitute testers for color vision, which may not include some commercially available vision testing machines. For an approved list, see Item, 52. Color Vision.

Examination Techniques:

1. Near visual acuity and intermediate visual acuity, if the latter is required, are determined for each eye separately and for both eyes together. Test values are recorded both with and without corrective glasses/lenses when either are worn or required to meet the standards. If the applicant is unable to meet the intermediate acuity standard unaided, then he/she is tested using each of the corrective lenses or glasses otherwise needed by that person to meet distant and/or near visual acuity standards. If the aided acuity meets the standard using any of the lenses or glasses, the findings are recorded, and the certificate appropriately limited. If an applicant has no lenses that bring intermediate and/or near visual acuity to the required standards, or better, in each eye, no certificate may be issued, and the applicant is referred to an eye specialist for appropriate visual evaluation and correction.

2. FAA Form 8500-1, Near Vision Acuity Test Chart, dated April 1993, should be used as follows:

   a. The examination is conducted in a well-lighted room with the source of light behind the applicant.

   b. The applicant holds the chart 16 inches (near) and 32 inches (intermediate) from the eyes in a position that will provide uniform illumination. To ensure that the chart is held at exactly 16 inches or 32 inches from the eyes, a string of that length may be attached to the chart.

   c. Each eye is tested separately, with the other eye covered. Both eyes are then tested together.

   d. The smallest type correctly read with each eye separately and both eyes together is recorded in linear value. In performing the test using FAA Form 8500-1, the level of visual acuity will be recorded as the line of smallest type the applicant reads accurately. The applicant should be allowed no more than two misread letters on any line.

   e. Common errors:

      1. Inadequate illumination of the test chart.
      2. Failure to hold the chart the specified distance from the eye.
      3. Failure to ensure that the untested eye is covered.
      4. Failure to determine uncorrected and corrected acuity when the applicant wears glasses.

   f. Practical Test. At the bottom of FAA Form 8500-1 is a section for Aeronautical Chart Reading. Letter types and charts are reproduced from aeronautical charts in their actual size.

This may be used when a borderline condition exists at the certifiable limits of an applicant's vision. If successfully completed, a favorable certification action may be taken.

3. Acceptable substitute equipment may be used. Directions furnished by the manufacturer or distributor should be followed when using the acceptable substitute devices for the above testing.

III. Aerospace Medical Disposition

When correcting glasses are required to meet the near and intermediate vision standards, an appropriate limitation will be placed on the medical certificate. Contact lenses that correct only for near or intermediate visual acuity are not considered acceptable for aviation duties.

If the applicant meets the uncorrected near or intermediate vision standard of 20/40, but already uses spectacles that correct the vision better than 20/40, it is recommended that the Examiner enter the limitation for near or intermediate vision corrective glasses on the certificate.

For all classes, the appropriate wording for the near vision limitation is:

HOLDER SHALL POSSESS GLASSES THAT CORRECT FOR NEAR VISION

Possession only is required, because it may be hazardous to have distant vision obscured by the continuous wearing of reading glasses.

For first- and second-class, the appropriate wording for combined near and intermediate vision limitation is:

HOLDER SHALL POSSESS GLASSES THAT CORRECT FOR NEAR AND INTERMEDIATE VISION

For multiple defective distant, near, and intermediate visual acuity when unifocal glasses or contact lenses are used and correct all, the appropriate limitation is:

HOLDER SHALL WEAR CORRECTIVE LENSES

For multiple vision defects involving distance and/or near and/or intermediate visual acuity when more than one set of lenses is required to correct for all vision defects, the appropriate limitation is:

HOLDER SHALL WEAR LENSES THAT CORRECT FOR DISTANT VISION AND POSSESS GLASSES THAT CORRECT FOR NEAR AND INTERMEDIATE VISION

ITEM 52. Color Vision

52. Color Vision	
☐	Pass
☐	Fail

I. Code of Federal Regulations

First- and Second-Classes: 14 CFR 67.103(c) and 67.203(c)

(c) Color vision: Ability to perceive those colors necessary for the safe performance of airman duties.

Third-Class: 14 CFR 67.303(c)

(c) Color vision: Ability to perceive those colors necessary for the safe performance of airman duties.

II. Examination Equipment and Techniques

The following equipment and techniques apply only to airmen. **Not all tests approved for airmen are acceptable for air traffic controllers (FAA employee 2152 series and contract tower air traffic controllers).**

For ATCS information, see the end of this section or contact a Regional Flight Surgeon.

EQUIPMENT	TEST	EDITION	PLATES
Pseudoisochromatic plates	Test book should be held 30" from applicant Plates should be illuminated by at least 20' candles, preferably by a Macbeth Easel Lamp or a Verilux True Color Light (F15T8VLX) Only three seconds are allowed for the applicant to interpret and respond to a given plate		
American Optical Company [AOC]		1965	1-15
AOC-HRR		2nd	1-11
Richmond-HRR		4th	5-24
Dvorine		2nd	1-15
Ishihara		14 Plate	1-11
		24 Plate	1-15
		38 Plate	1-21
Richmond, 15-plates		1983	1-15

Acceptable Substitutes: (May be used following the directions accompanying the instruments) Farnsworth Lantern; OPTEC 900 Color Vision Test; Keystone Orthoscope; Keystone Telebinocular; OPTEC 2000 Vision Tester (Model Nos. 2000 PM, 2000 PAME, and 2000 PI); OPTEC 2500; Titmus Vision Tester; Titmus 2 Vision Tester (Model Nos. T2A and T2S); Titmus i400.

III. Aerospace Medical Disposition

The following criteria apply only to airmen. **Not all tests approved for airmen are acceptable for air traffic controllers (FAA employee 2152 series and contract tower air traffic controllers). For ATCS information, see the end of this section or contact a Regional Flight Surgeon.**

An applicant meets the color vision standard if he/she passes any of the color vision tests listed in Examination Techniques, Item 52. Color Vision. If an applicant fails any of these tests, inform the applicant of the option of taking any of the other acceptable color vision tests listed in Item 52. Color Vision Examination Equipment and Techniques before requesting the Specialized Operational Medical Tests in Section D below.

Inform the applicant that if he/she takes and fails any component of the Specialized Operational Medical Tests in Section D, then he/she will not be permitted to take any of the remaining listed office-based color vision tests in Examination Techniques, Item 52. Color Vision as an attempt to remove any color vision limits or restrictions on their airman medical certificate. That pathway is no longer an option to the airman, and no new result will be considered.

An applicant does not meet the color vision standard if testing reveals:

A. All Classes

1. AOC (1965 edition) pseudoisochromatic plates: seven or more errors on plates 1-15.
2. AOC-HRR (second edition): Any error in test plates 7-11. Because the first 4 plates in the test book are for demonstration only, test plate 7 is actually the eleventh plate in the book. (See instruction booklet.)
3. Dvorine pseudoisochromatic plates (second edition, 15 plates): seven or more errors on plates 1-15.
4. Ishihara pseudoisochromatic plates: Concise 14-plate edition: six or more errors on plates 1-11; the 24-plate edition: seven or more errors on plates 1-15; the 38-plate edition: nine or more errors on plates 1-21.
5. Richmond (1983 edition) pseudoisochromatic plates: seven or more errors on plates 1-15.
6. OPTEC 900 Vision Tester and Farnsworth Lantern test: an average of more than one error per series of nine color pairs in series 2 and 3. (See instruction booklet.)

7. Titmus Vision Tester, Titmus 2 Vision Tester, Titmus i400, OPTEC 2000 Vision Tester, Keystone Orthoscope, or Keystone View Telebinocular: any errors in the six plates.

8. LKC Technologies, Inc., APT-5 Color Vision Tester: The letter must be correctly identified in at least two of the three presentations of each test condition. (See APT-5 screening chart for FAA-related testing in instruction booklet.)

9. Richmond-HRR, 4th edition: two or more errors on plates 5-24. Plates 1-4 are for demonstration only; plates 5-10 are screening plates; and plates 11-24 are diagnostic plates.

B. Certificate Limitation. If an applicant fails to meet the color vision standard as interpreted above, but is otherwise qualified, the Examiner must issue a medical certificate bearing the limitation:

NOT VALID FOR NIGHT FLYING OR BY COLOR SIGNAL CONTROL

C. The color vision screening tests above (Section A) are not to be used for the purpose of removing color vision limits/restrictions from medical certificates of airmen who have failed the Specialized Operational Medical Tests below (Section D). See bold paragraph in the introduction of this section (above).

D. Specialized Operational Medical Tests for Applicants Who Do Not Meet the Standard. Applicants who fail the color vision screening test as listed, but desire an airman medical certificate without the color vision limitation, may be given, upon request, an opportunity to take and pass additional operational color perception tests. If the airman passes the operational color vision perception test(s), then he/she will be issued a Letter of Evidence (LOE).

- The operational tests are determined by the class of medical certificate requested. The request should be in writing and directed to AMCD or RFS. See NOTE for description of the operational color perception tests.

- Applicants for a third-class medical certificate need only take the Operational Color Vision Test (OCVT).

- The applicant is permitted to take the OVCT only once during the day. If the applicant fails, he/she may request to take the OVCT at night. If the applicant elects to take the OCVT at night, he/she may take it only once.

- For an upgrade to first- or second-class medical certificate, the applicant must first pass the OCVT during daylight and then pass the color vision Medical Flight Test (MFT). If the applicant fails the OCVT during the day, he/she will not be allowed to apply for an upgrade to First- or Second-Class certificate. If the applicant fails the color vision MFT, he/she is not permitted to upgrade to a first- or second-class certificate.

E. An LOE may restrict an applicant to a third-class medical certificate. Airmen shall not be issued a medical certificate of higher class than indicated on the LOE. Exercise care in reviewing an LOE before issuing a medical certificate to an airman.

F. Color Vision Correcting Lens (e.g. X-Chrom). Such lenses are unacceptable to the FAA as a means for correcting a pilot's color vision deficiencies.

G. Any tests not specifically listed above are unacceptable methods of testing for FAA medical certificate. Examples of unacceptable tests include, but are not limited to, the OPTEC 5000 Vision Tester (color vision portion), "Farnsworth Lantern *Flashlight*," "yarn tests," and AME-administered aviation Signal Light Gun test (AME office use is prohibited).

NOTE: An applicant for a third-class airman medical certificate who has defective color vision and desires an airman medical certificate without the color vision limitation must demonstrate the ability to pass an Operational Color Vision Test (OCVT) during the day. The OCVT consists of the following:
1. A Signal Light Test (SLT): Identify in a timely manner aviation red, green, and white
2. Aeronautical chart reading: Read and correctly interpret in a timely manner aeronautical charts, including print in various sizes, colors, and typefaces; conventional markings in several colors; and, terrain colors

An applicant for a first- or second- class airman medical certificate who has defective color vision and desires an airman medical certificate without the color vision limitation must first demonstrate the ability to pass the OCVT during the day (as above) and then must pass a color vision Medical Flight Test (MFT). The color vision MFT is performed in the aircraft, including in-flight testing. It consists of the following:

1. Read and correctly interpret in a timely manner aviation instruments or displays
2. Recognize terrain and obstructions in a timely manner
3. Visually identify in a timely manner the location, color, and significance of aeronautical lights such as, but not limited to, lights of other aircraft in the vicinity, runway lighting systems, etc.

Applicants who take and pass both the OCVT during the day and the color vision MFT will be given a letter of evidence (LOE) valid for all classes of medical certificates and will have no limitation or comment made on the certificate regarding color vision as they meet the standard for all classes. Applicants who take and pass only the OCVT during the day will be given an LOE valid only for third-class medical certificate.

An applicant who fails the SLT portion of the OCVT during daylight hours may repeat the test at night. Should the airman pass the SLT at night, the restriction:

NOT VALID FOR FLIGHT DURING DAYLIGHT HOURS BY COLOR SIGNAL CONTROL

will be placed on the replacement medical certificate. The airman must have taken the daylight hours test first and failed prior to taking the night test.

Color Vision Testing Flowchart

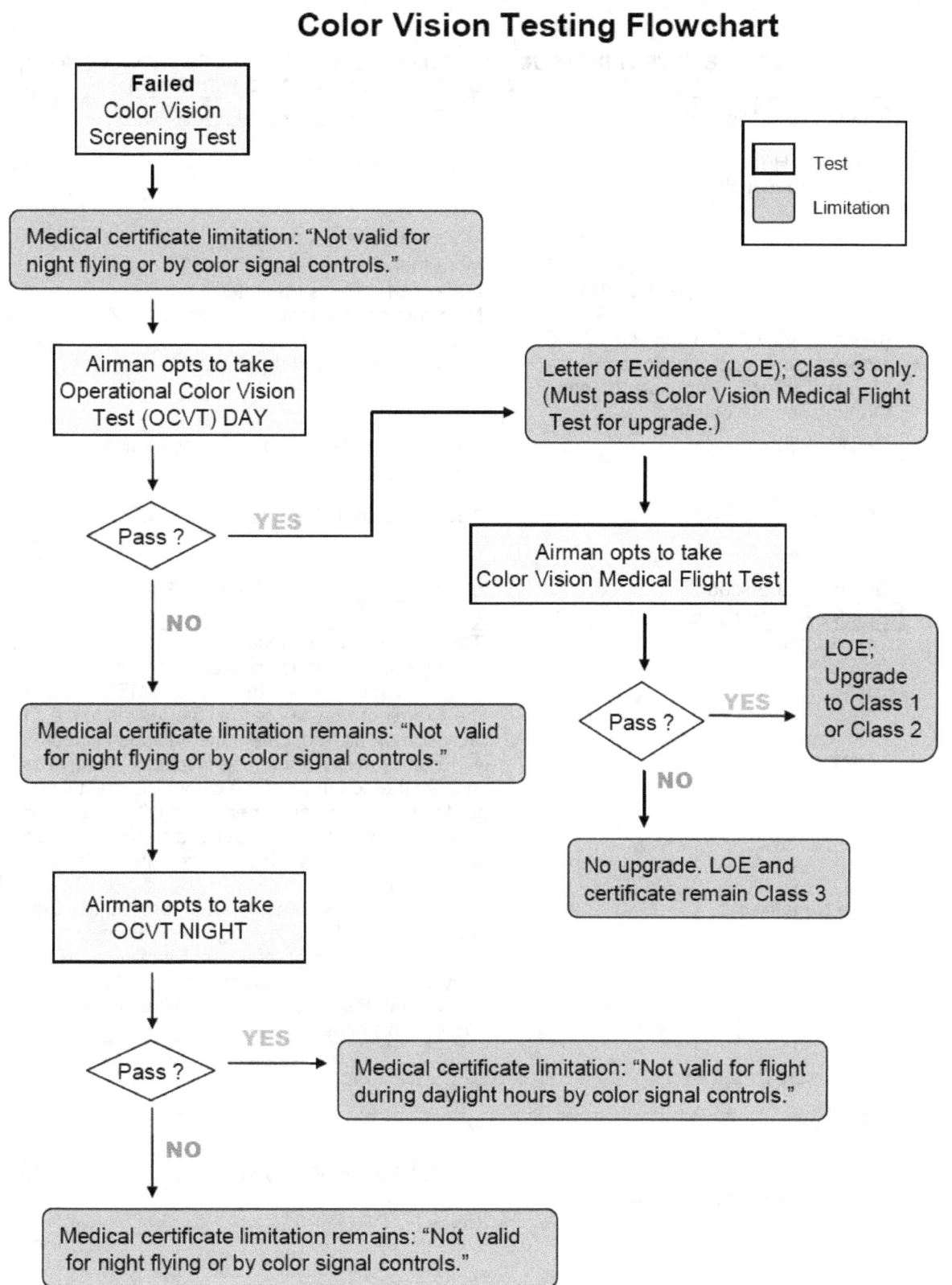

ACCEPTABLE TEST INSTRUMENTS FOR COLOR VISION SCREENING OF ATCS
(FAA EMPLOYEE 2152 SERIES and CONTRACT TOWER ATCSs)

Color Vision Test	Does not meet the standard (fails) if:	Supplier
Richmond-HRR, 4th edition	Any error on plates 5-10	Richmond Products
All Ishihara test plates approved for airmen:		Ishihara
14-Plate (plates 1-11)	More than 6 errors on plates 1-11	
24-Plate (plates 1-15)	More than 2 errors on plates 1-15	
38-Plate (plates 1-21)	More than 4 errors on plates 1-21	
Keystone View Telebinocular	No errors on the 6 total trials on plates 4 and 5	Keystone View
Titmus testers approved for airmen: Titmus, Titmus II, Titmus 2a/2s (one is manual, one is electronic)	Any errors on any of the 6 plates	Titmus
OPTEC 2000	Any errors on any of the 6 Stereo Optical Co., Inc., plates	Stereo Optical Co., Inc.
AOC-HRR, 2nd, 1-11	Any errors on plates 5-10	Richmond Products
Dvorine 2nd Edition	More than 2 errors on plates 1-15	Richmond Products
Special Instructions		
Test Administration	The Examiner must document the color vision test instrument used, version, answer sheet with the actual subject responses and the score. If MEDExpress is used the examiner may fax or mail the results to the Flight Surgeon or may document the findings in block 60.	
AME Office Inspection	AME office inspections: The inspector must visually inspect the condition of the color vision test instrument, for fading, finger prints, pen or pencil smudges; and lights used. Only a Macbeth Easel or a Verilux True Daylight Illuminator (F15T8VLX) are acceptable. Room lights must be off.	
False Negatives	Any test device with a restricted test set, like the Titmus testers, generally have a high false alarm test. If a disproportionally high number of subjects are failing, it may be necessary to review the acceptability of that test instrument. Regional Medical Offices are expected to monitor this situation.	

UNACCEPTABLE TEST INSTRUMENTS FOR COLOR VISION SCREENING OF ATCS
(FAA EMPLOYEE 2152 SERIES and CONTRACT TOWER ATCSs)

AOC-PIP	Mast	Stereo-Optic
Bausch & Lomb Vision Tester	OPTEC 900, 2500*, 5000*	Titmus i400*
D-15	Prism	Vision Chart - color letters
FALANT	Richmond-HRR Versions 2 and 3	
H-O Chart	Schilling	

ITEM 53. Field of Vision

53. Field of Vision	
☐ Normal	☐ Abnormal

I. Code of Federal Regulations

First- and Second-Classes: 14 CFR 67.103(d) and 67.203(d)

(d) Field of Vision: Normal

Third-Class: 14 CFR 67.303(d)

(d) Field of Vision: No acute or chronic pathological condition of either eye or adnexa that interferes with the proper function of an eye, that may reasonably be expected to progress to that degree, or that may reasonably be expected to be aggravated by flying.

II. Examination Equipment and Techniques

1. Fifty-inch square black matte surface wall target with center white fixation point; 2 millimeter white test object on black-handled holder:

    1. The applicant should be seated 40 inches from the target.

    2. An occluder should be placed over the applicant's right eye.

    3. The applicant should be instructed to keep the left eye focused on the fixation point.

    4. The white test object should be moved from the outside border of the wall target toward the point of fixation on each of the eight 4-degree radials.

    5. The result should be recorded on a worksheet as the number of inches from the fixation point at which the applicant first identifies the white target on each radial.

    6. The test should be repeated with the applicant's left eye occluded and the right eye focusing on the fixation point.

2. Alternative Techniques:

    a. A standard perimeter may be used in place of the above procedure. With this method, any significant deviation from normal field configuration will require evaluation by an eye specialist.

b. Direct confrontation. This is the least acceptable alternative since this tests for peripheral vision and only grossly for field size and visual defects. The Examiner, standing in front of the applicant, has the applicant look at the Examiner's nose while advancing two moving fingers from slightly behind and to the side of the applicant in each of the four quadrants. Any significant deviation from normal requires ophthalmological evaluation.

III. Aerospace Medical Disposition

A. Ophthalmological Consultations.

If an applicant fails to identify the target in any presentation at a distance of less than 23 inches from the fixation point, an eye specialist's evaluation must be requested. This is a requirement for all classes of certification. The Examiner should provide FAA Form 8500-14, Ophthalmological Evaluation for Glaucoma, for use by the ophthalmologist if glaucoma is suspected.

B. Glaucoma.

The FAA may grant an Authorization under the special issuance section of part 67 (14 CFR 67.401) on an individual basis. The Examiner can facilitate FAA review by obtaining a report of Ophthalmological Evaluation for Glaucoma (FAA Form 8500-14) from a treating or evaluating ophthalmologist.

NOTE: See AASI for History of Glaucoma

If considerable disturbance in night vision is documented, the FAA may limit the medical certificate: NOT VALID FOR NIGHT FLYING

C. Other Pathological Conditions.

See **Items 31-34.**

ITEM 54. Heterophoria

54. Heterophoria 20' (in prism diopters)	Esophoria	Exophoria	Right Hyperphoria	Left Hyperphoria

I. Code of Federal Regulations

First- and Second-Classes: 14 CFR 67.103(f) and 67.203(f)

(f) Bifoveal fixation and vergence-phoria relationship sufficient to prevent a break in fusion under conditions that may reasonably be expected to occur in performing airman duties. Tests for the factors named in this paragraph are not required except for persons found to have more than 1 prism diopter of hyperphoria, 6 prism diopters of esophoria, or 6 prism diopters of exophoria. If any of these values are exceeded, the Federal Air Surgeon may require the person to be examined by a qualified eye specialist to determine if there is bifoveal fixation and an adequate vergence-phoria relationship. However, if otherwise eligible, the person is issued a medical certificate pending the results of the examination.

Third-Class: No Standards

II. Examination Equipment and Techniques

Equipment:

1. Red Maddox rod with handle.
2. Horizontal prism bar with graduated prisms beginning with one prism diopter and increasing in power to at least eight prism diopters.
3. Acceptable substitutes: any commercially available visual acuities and heterophoria testing devices.

   There are specific approved substitute testers for color vision, which may not include some commercially available vision testing machines. For an approved list, See Item, 52. Color Vision.

Examination Techniques:

Test procedures to be used accompany the instruments. If the Examiner needs specific instructions for use of the horizontal prism bar and red Maddox rod, these may be obtained from a RFS.

III. Aerospace Medical Disposition

1. First- and second-class: If an applicant exceeds the heterophoria standards (1 prism diopter of hyperphoria, 6 prism diopters of esophoria, or 6 prism diopters of exophoria), but shows no evidence of diplopia or serious eye pathology and all other aspects of the examination are favorable, the Examiner should not withhold or deny the medical certificate. The applicant should be advised that the FAA may require further examination by a qualified eye specialist.

2. Third-class: Applicants for a third-class certificate are not required to undergo heterophoria testing. However, if an applicant has strabismus or a history of diplopia, the Examiner should defer issuance of a certificate and forward the application to the AMCD. If the applicant wishes further consideration, the Examiner can help expedite FAA review by providing the applicant with a copy of FAA Form 8500-7, Report of Eye Evaluation.

ITEM 55. Blood Pressure

55. Blood Pressure		
	Systolic	Diastolic
(Sitting mm of Mercury)		

I. Code of Federal Regulations

All Classes: 14 CFR 67.113(b)(c), 67.213(b)(c), and 67.313(b)(c)

(b). No other organic, functional, or structural disease, defect, or limitation that the Federal Air Surgeon, based on the case history and appropriate, qualified medical judgment relating to the condition involved, finds -

(1). Makes the person unable to safely perform the duties or exercise the privileges of the airman certificate applied for or held; or

(2). May reasonably be expected, for the maximum duration of the airman medical certificate applied for or held, to make the person unable to perform those duties or exercise those privileges.

(c). No medication or other treatment that the Federal Air Surgeon, based on the case history and appropriate, qualified medical judgment relating to the medication or other treatment involved finds -

(1). Makes the person unable to safely perform the duties or exercise the privileges of the airman certificate applied for or held; or

(2). May reasonably be expected, for the maximum duration of the airman medical certificate applied for or held, to make the person unable to perform those duties or exercise those privileges.

Measurement of blood pressure is an essential part of the FAA medical certification examination. The average blood pressure while sitting should not exceed 155 mm mercury systolic and 95 mm mercury diastolic maximum pressure for all classes. A medical assessment is specified for all applicants who need or use antihypertensive medication to control blood pressure. (See Section III. B. below.)

II. Examination Techniques

In accordance with accepted clinical procedures, routine blood pressure should be taken with the applicant in the seated position. An applicant should not be denied or deferred first-, second-, or third-class certification unless subsequent recumbent blood pressure readings exceed those contained in this Guide. Any conditions that may adversely affect the validity of the blood pressure reading should be noted.

III. Aerospace Medical Disposition

A. Examining Options

1. An applicant whose pressure does not exceed 155 mm mercury systolic and 95 mm mercury diastolic maximum pressure, who has not used antihypertensive medication for 30 days, and who is otherwise qualified should be issued a medical certificate by the Examiner.

2. An applicant whose blood pressure is slightly elevated beyond the FAA specified limits, may, at the Examiner's discretion, have a series of 3 daily readings over a 7-day period. If the indication of hypertension remains, even if it is mild or intermittent, the Examiner should defer certification and transmit the application to the AMCD with a note of explanation.

   The Examiner must defer issuance of a medical certificate to any applicant whose hypertension has not been evaluated, who uses unacceptable medications, whose medical status is unclear, whose hypertension is uncontrolled, who manifests significant adverse effects of medication, or whose certification has previously been specifically reserved to the FAA.

B. Initial and Followup Evaluation for Hypertensives Under Treatment -
   See Hypertension Protocol

ITEM 56. Pulse

56. Pulse (Resting)

The medical standards do not specify pulse rates that, *per se*, are disqualifying for medical certification. These tests are used, however, to determine the status and responsiveness of the cardiovascular system. Abnormal pulse rates may be reason to conduct additional cardiovascular system evaluations.

II. Examination Techniques

The pulse rate is determined with the individual relaxed in a sitting position.

III. Aerospace Medical Disposition

If there is bradycardia, tachycardia, or arrhythmia, further evaluation is warranted and deferral may be indicated (see Item 36., Heart). A cardiac evaluation may be needed to determine the applicant's qualifications. Temporary stresses or fever may, at times, result in abnormal pulse readings. If the Examiner believes this to be the case, the applicant should be given a few days to recover and then be retested. If this is not possible, the Examiner should defer issuance, pending further evaluation.

ITEM 57. Urine Test

57. Urine Test (if abnormal, give results)		Albumin	Sugar
☐ Normal	☐ Abnormal		

I. Code of Federal Regulations

All Classes: 14 CFR 67.113(a)(b), 67.213(a)(b), and 67.313(a)(b)

(a) No established medical history or clinical diagnosis of diabetes mellitus that requires insulin or any other hypoglycemic drug for control.

(b) No other organic, functional, or structural disease, defect, or limitation that the Federal Air Surgeon, based on the case history and appropriate, qualified medical judgment relating to the condition involved, finds –

(1) Makes the person unable to safely perform the duties or exercise the privileges of the airman certificate applied for or held; or

(2) May reasonably be expected, for the maximum duration of the airman

medical certificate applied for or held, to make the person unable to perform those duties or exercise those privileges.

II. Examination Techniques

Any standard laboratory procedures are acceptable for these tests.

III. Aerospace Medical Disposition

Glycosuria or proteinuria is cause for deferral of medical certificate issuance until additional studies determine the status of the endocrine and/or urinary systems. If the glycosuria has been determined not to be due to carbohydrate intolerance, the Examiner may issue the certificate. Trace or 1+ proteinuria in the absence of a history of renal disease is not cause for denial.

The Examiner may request additional urinary tests when they are indicated by history or examination. These should be reported on FAA Form 8500-8 or attached to the form as an addendum.

See **Item 48., General Systemic.**

ITEM 58. ECG

58. ECG (Date) MM	DD	YYYY

I. Code of Federal Regulations

First-Class: 14 CFR 67.111(b)(c)

(b) A person applying for first-class medical certification must demonstrate an absence of myocardial infarction and other clinically significant abnormality on electrocardiographic examination:

(1) At the first application after reaching the 35th birthday; and

(2) On an annual basis after reaching the 40th birthday.

(c) An ECG will satisfy a requirement of paragraph (b) of this section if it is dated no earlier than 60 days before the date of the application it is to accompany and was performed and transmitted according to acceptable standards and techniques.

Note: All applicants for certification may be required to provide ECGs when indicated by history or physical examination.

II. Examination Techniques

A. Date. The date of the most recent ECG shall be entered in Item 58 of FAA Form 8500-8 for all first-class applicants.

1. If a first-class applicant is due for a periodic ECG, the Examiner performs and transmits a current tracing according to established procedures. (See Section II. D. below).

   However, some applicants (such as airline transport pilots who are employed by air carriers with medical departments) may have their company transmit a current ECG directly to the FAA. The Examiner need not require such an applicant to undergo another ECG examination and, if the applicant is otherwise qualified, a medical certificate may be issued. The Examiner should attach a statement to FAA Form 8500-8 to verify that a tracing has been transmitted from another source. The date of that ECG should be entered in Item 58.

2. If a first-class applicant is not required to have a periodic ECG with the current examination, the Examiner should record the date of the preceding ECG in Item 58.

3. If a second- or third-class applicant gives a history of having had an electrocardiogram, the test and date may be entered in Item 59. More importantly, the Examiner should indicate in Item 60 of FAA Form 8500-8 the history and its significance, if any.

4. If the applicant provides no statement and refuses to have a current ECG submitted by the Examiner, the Examiner should defer issuance of the medical certificate. When an ECG is due but is not submitted, the FAA will not affirm the applicant's eligibility for medical certification until the requested ECG has been received and interpreted as being within normal limits. Failure to respond to FAA requests for a required current ECG will result in denial of certification.

B. Currency

1. In order to meet regulatory requirements, a first-class applicant's periodic ECG must have been performed and transmitted within 60 days prior to the date of the first-class application (FAA Form 8500-8). The AMCD verifies currency of all periodic ECGs.

2. There is no provision for issuance of a first-class medical certificate based upon a promise that an ECG will be obtained at a future date. In such circumstances, the Examiner should defer issuance and transmit the completed FAA Form 8500-8 to the AMCD

C. Interpretation

1. All ECGs required to establish eligibility for medical certification must be forwarded for interpretation to the Manager of the AMCD. This does not preclude submission of an interpretation by or through the Examiner.

2. Interpretation is accomplished by the staff and consultant cardiologists at the AMCD. Abnormalities are investigated to determine their significance, if any.

D. Technique and Reporting Format for Required ECGs on First-class Applicants

The method for recording and transmitting ECGs is by digital electronic data transfer by the Examiner to the AMCD. Senior Examiners who perform first-class medical examinations are required to have access to this capability.

International Examiners who submit ECGs should use the following format for preparation and submission:

1. See FAA Form 8065-1, Instructions for Preparation and Submittal of Electrocardiogram. However, the FAA also will accept 3-channel or 12-channel strips uncut or mounted on standard mounting paper. The following steps are essential to expedite processing of these tracings:

   a. All leads must be properly identified.

   b. Applicant and Examiner identification must be complete and the tracing must be dated.

2. Such hard-copy ECGs are microfilmed for permanent retention in the AMCD. Only tracings that can be microfilmed are acceptable.

3. Provide a Resting tracing. Tracings must be stapled to the ECG report form to ensure that all leads are appropriately coded and interpreted.

APPLICATION REVIEW

Items 59-64 of FAA Form 8500-8

ITEMS 59-64 of FAA Form 8500-8

This section provides guidance for the completion of Items 59-64 of the FAA Form 8500-8. The Examiner is responsible for conducting the examination. However, he or she may delegate to a qualified physician's assistant, nurse, aide, or laboratory assistant the testing required for Items 49-58. Regardless of who performs the tests, the Examiner is responsible for the accuracy of the findings, and this responsibility **may not** be delegated.

The medical history page of FAA Form 8500-8 must be completed and certified by the applicant or it will not appear in AMCS. After all routine evaluations and tests are completed, the Examiner should review FAA Form 8500-8. If the form is complete and accurate, the Examiner should add final comments, make qualification decision statements, and certify the examination.

ITEM 59. Other Tests Given

59. Other Tests Given

I. Code of Federal Regulations

All Classes: 14 CFR 67.413(a)(b)

(a) Whenever the Administrator finds that additional medical information or history is necessary to determine whether an applicant for or the holder of a medical certificate meets the medical standards for it, the Administrator requests that person to furnish that information or to authorize any clinic, hospital, physician, or other person to release to the Administrator all available information or records concerning that history. If the applicant or holder fails to provide the requested medical information or history or to authorize the release so requested, the Administrator may suspend, modify, or revoke all medical certificates the airman holds or may, in the case of an applicant, deny the application for an airman medical certificate.

(b) If an airman medical certificate is suspended or modified under paragraph (a) of this section, that suspension or modification remains in effect until the requested information, history, or authorization is provided to the FAA and until the Federal Air Surgeon determines whether the person meets the medical standards under this part.

II. Examination Techniques

Additional medical information may be furnished through additional history taking, further clinical examination procedures, and supplemental laboratory procedures.

On rare occasions, even surgical procedures such as biopsies may be indicated. As a designee of the FAA Administrator, the Examiner has limited authority to apply 14 CFR 67.413 in processing applications for medical certification. When an Examiner determines that there is a need for additional medical information, based upon history and findings, the Examiner is authorized to request prior hospital and outpatient records and to request supplementary examinations including laboratory testing and examinations by appropriate medical specialists. The Examiner should discuss the need with the applicant. The applicant should be advised of the types of additional examinations required and the type of medical specialist to be consulted. Responsibility for ensuring that these examinations are forwarded and that any charges or fees are paid will rest with the applicant. All reports should be forwarded to the AMCD, unless otherwise directed (such as by a RFS).

Whenever, in the Examiner's opinion, medical records are necessary to evaluate an applicant's medical fitness, the Examiner should request that the applicant sign an authorization for the Release of Medical Information. The Examiner should forward this authorization to the custodian of the applicant's records so that the information contained in the record may be obtained for attachment to the report of medical examination.

ITEM 60. Comments On History and Findings

Comments on all positive history or medical examination findings must be reported by **Item Number**. Item 60 provides the Examiner an opportunity to report observations and/or findings that are not asked for on the application form. Concern about the applicant's behavior, abnormal situations arising during the examination, unusual findings, unreported history, and other information thought germane to aviation safety should be reported in Item 60. The Examiner should record name, dosage, frequency, and purpose for all currently used medications.

If possible, all ancillary reports such as consultations, ECGs, x-ray release forms, and hospital or other treatment records should be attached. If the delay for those items would exceed 14 days, the Examiner should forward all available data to the AMCD, with a note specifying what additional information is being prepared for submission at a later date.

If there are no significant medical history items or abnormal physical findings, the Examiner should indicate this by checking the appropriate block.

ITEM 61. Applicant's Name

Item 61. Applicant's Name

The legal name applicant's name should be entered.

ITEM 62. Has Been Issued

Item 62. Has Been Issued	☐ Medical Certificate	☐ Medical & Student Pilot Certificate
☐	No Medical Certificate Issued	Deferred for Further Evaluation
☐	Has Been Denied	Letter of Denial Issued (Copy Attached)

The Examiner must check the proper box to indicate if the Medical Certificate, FAA Form 8500-9 (white), or Medical Certificate and Student Pilot Certificate, FAA Form 8420-2 (yellow), has been issued. If neither form has been issued, the Examiner must indicate denial or deferral by checking one of the two lower boxes. If denied, a copy of the Examiner's Letter of Denial, should be forwarded to the AMCD.

A. Applicant's Refusal. When advised by an Examiner that further examination and/or medical records are needed, the applicant may elect not to proceed. The Examiner should note this on FAA Form 8500-8. No certificate should be issued, and the Examiner should forward the application form to the AMCD, even if the application is incomplete.

B. Anticipated Delay. When the Examiner anticipates a delay of more than 14 days in obtaining records or reports concerning additional examinations, the completed FAA Form 8500-8 should be transmitted to the AMCD with a note stating that additional information will follow. No medical certificate should be issued.

C. Issuance. When the Examiner receives all the supplemental information requested and finds that the applicant meets all the FAA medical standards for the class sought, the Examiner should issue a medical certificate.

D. Deferral. If upon receipt of the information the Examiner finds there is a need for even more information or there is uncertainty about the significance of the findings, certification should be deferred. The Examiner's concerns should be noted on FAA Form 8500-8 and the application transmitted to the AMCD for further consideration.

If the applicant decides at this point to abandon the application for a medical certificate, the Examiner should also note this on FAA Form 8500-8 and mail the incomplete form to the AMCD. An incomplete FAA Form 8500-8 should not be transmitted to the AMCD for further consideration.

E. Denial. When the Examiner concludes that the applicant is clearly ineligible for certification, the applicant should be denied, using the AME Letter of Denial. Use of this form will provide the applicant with the reason for the denial and with appeal rights and procedures. (See **General Information, 4**. Medical Certification Decision Making)

ITEM 63. Disqualifying Defects

The Examiner must check the "Disq" box on the Comments Page beside any disqualifying defect. Comments or discussion of specific observations or findings may be reported in **Item 60**. If all comments cannot fit in Item 60, the Examiner may submit additional information on a plain sheet of paper and include the applicant's full name, date of birth, signature, any appropriate identifying numbers (PI, MID or SSN), and the date of the exam.

If the Examiner denies the applicant, the Examiner must issue a Letter of Denial, to the applicant, and report the issuance of the denial in Item 60.

ITEM 64. Medical Examiner's Declaration

- The FAA designates specific individuals as Examiners and this status may not be delegated to staff or to a physician who may be covering the designee's practice.

- Before transmitting to AMCD, the Examiner must certify the exam and enter all appropriate information including his or her AME serial number.

DISEASE PROTOCOLS

PROTOCOLS

The following lists the Guide for Aviation Medical Examiners Disease Protocols, and course of action that should be taken by the Examiner as defined by aeromedical decision considerations.

- ALLERGIES, SEVERE
- BINOCULAR MULTIFOCAL AND ACCOMMODATING DEVICES
- CARDIAC TRANSPLANT
- CARDIOVASCULAR EVALUATION
- CONDUCTIVE KERATOPLASTY
- CORONARY HEART DISEASE
- INSULIN TREATED DIABETES MELLITUS - Type I or Type II
- MEDICATION CONTROLLED DIABETES MELLITUS - Type II
- DIET CONTROLLED DIABETES MELLITUS and METABOLIC SYNDROME
- GRADED EXERCISE STRESS TEST REQUIREMENTS
- HUMAN IMMUNODEFICIENCY VIRUS (HIV)
- HYPERTENSION
- IMPLANTED PACEMAKER
- MEDICATION CONTROLLED METABOLIC SYNDROME (Glucose Intolerance, Impaired Glucose Tolerance, Impaired Fasting Glucose, Insulin Resistance, and Pre-Diabetes)
- MUSCULOSKELETAL EVALUATION
- PEPTIC ULCER
- RENAL TRANSPLANT
- SUBSTANCES of DEPENDENCE/ABUSE (Drugs and Alcohol)
- THROMBOEMBOLIC DISEASE
- VALVE REPLACEMENT

PROTOCOL FOR ALLERGIES, SEVERE

In the case of severe allergies, the Examiner should deny or defer certification and provide a report to the Aerospace Medical Certification Division, AAM-300, that details the period and duration of symptoms and the nature and dosage of drugs used for treatment and/or prevention.

PROTOCOL FOR BINOCULAR MULTIFOCAL AND ACCOMMODATING DEVICES

This Protocol establishes the authority for the Examiner to issue an airman medical certificate to binocular applicants using multifocal or accommodating ophthalmic devices.

Devices acceptable for aviation-related duties must be FDA approved and include:

Intraocular Lenses (multifocal or accommodating intraocular lens implants)
Bifocal/Multifocal contact lenses

Examiners may issue as outlined below:

- Adaptation period before certification:
  - Surgical lens implantation – minimum 3 months post-operative
  - Contact lenses (bifocal or multifocal) – minimum one month of use

- Must provide a report to include the FAA Form 8500-7, Report of Eye Evaluation, from the operating surgeon or the treating eye specialist. This report must attest to stable visual acuity and refractive error, absence of significant side effects/complications, need of medications, and freedom from any glare, flares or other visual phenomena that could affect visual performance and impact aviation safety

- The following visual standards, as required for each class, must be met for each eye:

Distant   **First- and Second-Class**
20/20 or better in each eye separately, with or without correction

                        Third-Class
20/40 or better in each eye separately, with or without correction

Near   **All Classes**
20/40 or better in each eye separately (Snellen equivalent), with or without correction, as measured at 16 inches

Intermediate **First- and Second-Class**
20/40 or better in each eye separately (Snellen equivalent), with or without correction at age 50 and over, as measured at 32 inches

                        Third-Class
No requirement

Note: The above does not change the current certification policy on the use of monofocal non-accommodating intraocular lenses.

PROTOCOL FOR CARDIAC TRANSPLANT

The Examiner must defer issuance. Issuance is considered for Third-class applicants only. FAA Cardiology Panel will review. Applicants found qualified will be required to provide annual followup evaluations. All studies must be performed within 30 days of application.

Requirements for consideration:

- A 1 year recovery period shall elapse after the cardiac transplant before consideration

- A current report from the treating transplant cardiologist regarding the status of the cardiac transplant, including all pre- and post-operative reports. A statement regarding functional capacity, modifiable cardiovascular risk factors, and prognosis for incapacitation

- Current blood chemistries (fasting blood sugar, hemoglobin A1C concentration, and blood lipid profile to include total cholesterol, HDL, LDL, and triglycerides), within 30 days

- Any tests performed or deemed necessary by all treating physicians (e.g., myocardial biopsy)

- Coronary Angiogram

- Graded Exercise Stress Test (see disease protocol) and stress echocardiogram

- A current 24-hour Holter monitor evaluation to include selective representative tracings

- Complete documentation of all rejection history, whether treated or not; include hospital records and reports of any tests done

- A complete history regarding any infectious process

- All complete history regarding any malignancy

- List of all present medications and dosages, including side effects.

It is the responsibility of each applicant to provide the medical information required to determine his/her eligibility for airman medical certification. A medical release form may help in obtaining the necessary information. Please ensure full name appears on any reports or correspondence.

All information shall be forwarded in <u>one mailing</u> to either:

Medical Appeals Section, AAM-313
Aerospace Medical Certification Division
Federal Aviation Administration
Post Office Box 26080
Oklahoma City OK 73125-9914

Medical Appeals Section, AAM-313
Aerospace Medical Certification Division
Federal Aviation Administration
6700 S MacArthur Blvd., Room B-13
Oklahoma City OK 73169AASI FOR

PROTOCOL FOR CARDIOVASCULAR EVALUATION

A current cardiovascular evaluation must include:

- An assessment of personal and family medical history

- Clinical cardiac and general physical examination

- An assessment and statement regarding the applicant's medications, functional capacity, modifiable cardiovascular risk factors

- Motivation for any necessary change

- Prognosis for incapacitation

- Blood chemistries (fasting blood sugar, current blood lipid profile to include total cholesterol, HDL, LDL, and triglycerides) performed within the last 90 days

PROTOCOL FOR CONDUCTIVE KERATOPLASTY

Conductive Keratoplasty (CK) is a refractive surgery procedure. It is acceptable for aeromedical certification, with Special Issuance, after review by the FAA.

The following criteria are necessary for initial certification:

- The airman is not qualified for six months post procedure

- The airman must provide all medical records related to the procedure

- A current status report by the surgical eye specialist with special note regarding complications of the procedure or the acquired monocularity, or vision complaints by the airman

- A current FAA Form 8500-7, Report of Eye Evaluation

- A medical flight test may be necessary (consult with the FAA)

- Annual followups by the surgical eye specialist

PROTOCOL FOR EVALUATION OF CORONARY HEART DISEASE

Myocardial infarction, angina pectoris, or other evidence of coronary heart disease are covered in this protocol. Reports and test results relating to the diagnosis in accordance with the attached protocol must be obtained and forwarded to the AMCD.

A. Requirements are for consideration for any class of airman medical certification.

    1. Recovery periods before consideration can be given for medical certification:

        a. 6 months: after angina, infarction, bypass surgery, angioplasty, stenting, rotoblation, or atherectomy

        b. 3 months: after ablation or valve repair

        c. None: after supraventricular tachycardia, atrial fibrillation, and syncope. NOTE: if any of these conditions required any cardiac intervention that is listed in subparagraphs a and b above, then the applicable waiting periods do apply.

    2. Hospital admission summary (history and physical), coronary catheterization report, and operative report regarding all cardiac events and procedures.

    3. A current cardiovascular evaluation must include an assessment of personal and family medical history; a clinical cardiac and general physical examination; an assessment and statement regarding the applicant's medications, functional capacity, modifiable cardiovascular risk factors, motivation for any necessary change, prognosis for incapacitation; and blood chemistries (fasting blood sugar and current blood lipid profile to include total cholesterol, HDL, LDL, and triglycerides).

    4. A current maximal GXT – See GXT Protocol.

    A **SPECT** myocardial perfusion exercise stress test using technetium agents and/or thallium may be required for consideration for any class if clinically indicated or the exercise stress test is abnormal by any of the usual parameters. The interpretive report and all **SPECT** images, preferably in black and white, must be submitted.

    NOTE: If cardiac catheterization and/or coronary angiography have been performed, all reports and the actual films (if films are requested) must be submitted for review. Copies should be made of all films as a safeguard against loss. Films should be labeled with the name of the applicant and a return address.

B. Additional requirements for first or unlimited* second-class medical certification. The following should be accomplished no sooner than 6-months post event:

1. Post-event coronary angiography. The application may be considered without post-event angiography but certification for first- and unlimited second-class is unlikely without it.

2. A maximal thallium exercise stress test (See A. 4).

3. The applicant should indicate if a lower class medical certificate is acceptable in the event ineligible for class sought.

C. Certification. Applicants found qualified for an airman medical certificate will be required to provide periodic followup cardiovascular evaluations including maximal stress testing. Additional diagnostic testing modalities, including radionuclide studies, may be required if indicated.

No consideration will be given for an Authorization of Special Issuance of a Medical Certificate until all the required data have been received. The use of the applicant's full name, date of birth, and social security number on all correspondence and reports will aid the agency in locating the proper file.

It is the responsibility of each applicant to provide the medical information required to determine his/her eligibility for airman medical certification. In order to expedite processing, it is suggested that the information be sent in ONE MAILING, when possible, to either:

Medical Appeals Section, AAM-313   Medical Appeals Section, AAM-313
Aerospace Medical Certification Division   Aerospace Medical Certification Division
Federal Aviation Administration   Federal Aviation Administration
Post Office Box 26080   6700 S MacArthur Blvd., Room B-13
Oklahoma City OK 73125-9914   Oklahoma City OK 73169

D. Coronary Intervention (CABG, Rotoblation, Atherectomy, PTCA, and STENT).

In addition, the applicant must provide the operative or procedure report if a STENT was implanted. The report must include make, manufacturer, and type of STENT, implant location(s), and length and diameter of each STENT.

*Limited second-class medical certificate refers to a second-class certificate with a functional limitation such as, "Not Valid for Carrying Passengers for Compensation or Hire", "Not Valid for Pilot in Command", "Valid Only When Serving as a Pilot Member of a Fully Qualified Two-Pilot Crew," etc.

PROTOCOL FOR INSULIN-TREATED
DIABETES MELLITUS - TYPE I & TYPE II

The FAA has established a policy that permits the special issuance medical certification of insulin-treated applicants for third-class medical certification. Consideration will be given only to those individuals who have been clinically stable on their current treatment regimen for a period of 6-months or more. Consideration is *not* being given for first- or second-class certification. Individuals certificated under this policy will be required to provide substantial documentation regarding their history of treatment, accidents related to their disease, and current medical status. If certificated, they will be required to adhere to stringent monitoring requirements and are prohibited from operating aircraft outside the United States. The following is a summary of the evaluation protocol and an outline of the conditions that the FAA will apply:

A. Initial Certification

   1. The applicant must have had no recurrent (two or more) episodes of hypoglycemia in the past 5 years and none in the preceding 1 year which resulted in loss of consciousness, seizure, impaired cognitive function or requiring intervention by another party, or occurring without warning (hypoglycemia unawareness).

   2. The applicant will be required to provide copies of all medical records as well as accident and incident records pertinent to their history of diabetes.

   3. A report of a complete medical examination preferably by a physician who specializes in the treatment of diabetes will be required. The report must include, as a minimum:

      a. Two measurements of glycosylated hemoglobin (total A_1 or A_{1c} concentration and the laboratory reference range), separated by at least 90 days. The most recent measurement must be no more than 90 days old.

      b. Specific reference to the applicant's insulin dosages and diet.

      c. Specific reference to the presence or absence of cerebrovascular, cardiovascular, or peripheral vascular disease or neuropathy.

      d. Confirmation by an eye specialist of the absence of clinically significant eye disease.

      e. Verification that the applicant has been educated in diabetes and its control and understands the actions that should be taken if complications, especially hypoglycemia, should arise. The examining physician must also verify that the applicant has the ability and willingness to properly monitor and manage his or her diabetes.

f. If the applicant is age 40 or older, a report, with ECG tracings, of a maximal graded exercise stress test.

g. The applicant shall submit a statement from his/her treating physician, Examiner, or other knowledgeable person attesting to the applicant's dexterity and ability to determine blood glucose levels using a recording glucometer.

NOTE: Student pilots may wish to ensure they are eligible for medical certification prior to beginning or resuming flight instruction or training. In order to serve as a pilot in command, you must have a valid medical certificate for the type of operation performed.

B. Subsequent Medical Certification

1. For documentation of diabetes management, the applicant will be required to carry and use a whole blood glucose measuring device with memory and must report to the FAA immediately any hypoglycemic incidents, any involvement in accidents that result in serious injury (whether or not related to hypoglycemia); and any evidence of loss of control of diabetes, change in treatment regimen, or significant diabetic complications. With any of these occurrences, the individual must cease flying until cleared by the FAA.

2. At 3-month intervals, the airman must be evaluated by the treating physician. This evaluation must include a general physical examination, review of the interval medical history, and the results of a test for glycosylated hemoglobin concentration. The physician must review the record of the airman's daily blood glucose measurements and comment on the results. The results of these quarterly evaluations must be accumulated and submitted annually unless there has been a change. (See No. 1 above - If there has been a change the individual must report the change(s) to the FAA and wait for an eligibility letter before resuming flight duties).

3. On an annual basis, the reports from the examining physician must include confirmation by an eye specialist of the absence of significant eye disease.

4. At the first examination after age 40 and at 5-year intervals, the report, with ECG tracings, of a maximal graded exercise stress test must be included in consideration of continued medical certification.

C. Monitoring and Actions Required During Flight Operations

To ensure safe flight, the insulin using diabetic airman must carry during flight a recording glucometer; adequate supplies to obtain blood samples; and an amount of rapidly absorbable glucose, in 10 gm portions, appropriate to the planned duration of the flight. The following actions shall be taken in connection with flight operations:

1. One-half hour prior to flight, the airman must measure the blood glucose concentration. If it is less than 100 mg/dl the individual must ingest an appropriate (not less than 10 gm) glucose snack and measure the glucose concentration one-half hour later. If the concentration is within 100 -- 300 mg/dl, flight operations may be undertaken. If less than 100, the process must be repeated; if over 300, the

flight must be canceled.

2. One hour into the flight, at each successive hour of flight, and within one half hour prior to landing, the airman must measure their blood glucose concentration. If the concentration is less than 100 mg/dl, a 20 gm glucose snack shall be ingested. If the concentration is 100 -- 300 mg/dl, no action is required. If the concentration is greater that 300 mg/dl, the airman must land at the nearest suitable airport and may not resume flight until the glucose concentration can be maintained in the 100 -- 300 mg/dl range. In respect to determining blood glucose concentrations during flight, the airman must use judgment in deciding whether measuring concentrations or operational demands of the environment (e.g., adverse weather, etc.) should take priority. In cases where it is decided that operational demands take priority, the airman must ingest a10 gm glucose snack and measure his or her blood glucose level 1 hour later. If measurement is not practical at that time, the airman must ingest a 20 gm glucose snack and land at the nearest suitable airport so that a determination of the blood glucose concentration may be made.

(Note: Insulin pumps are acceptable)

PROTOCOL FOR HISTORY OF MEDICATION-CONTROLLED (NON INSULIN) DIABETES MELLITUS – TYPE II

This protocol is used for all diabetic applicants treated with oral agents or incretin mimetic medications (such as exenatide), herein referred to as medication(s).

An applicant with a diagnosis of diabetes mellitus controlled by use of a medication may be considered by the FAA for an Authorization of a Special Issuance of a Medical Certificate (Authorization). Following initiation of medication treatment, a 60-day period must elapse prior to certification to assure stabilization, adequate control, and the absence of side effects or complications from the medication.

The initial Authorization decision is made by the AMCD and may not be made by the Examiner. An Examiner may re-issue a subsequent airman medical certificate under the provisions of the Authorization.

The initial Authorization determination will be made on the basis of a report from the treating physician. For favorable consideration, the report must contain a statement regarding the medication used, dosage, the absence or presence of side effects and clinically significant hypoglycemic episodes, and an indication of satisfactory control of the diabetes. The results of an A1C hemoglobin determination within the past 30 days must be included. Note must also be made of the presence of cardiovascular, neurological, renal, and/or ophthalmological disease. The presence of one or more of these associated diseases will not be, per se, disqualifying but the disease(s) must be carefully evaluated to determine any added risk to aviation safety.

Re-issuance of a medical certificate under the provisions of an Authorization will also be made on the basis of reports from the treating physician. The contents of the report must contain the same information required for initial issuance and specifically reference the presence or absence of satisfactory control, any change in the dosage or type of medication, and the presence or absence of complications or side effects from the medication. In the event of an adverse change in the applicant's diabetic status (poor control or complications or side effects from the medication), or the appearance of an associated systemic disease, an Examiner must defer the case with all documentation to the AMCD for consideration.

If, upon further review of the deferred case, AMCD decides that re-issuance is appropriate, the Examiner may again be given the authority to re-issue the medical certificate under the provisions of the Authorization based on data provided by the treating physician, including such information as may be required to assess the status of associated medical condition(s).

At a minimum, followup evaluation by the treating physician of the applicant's diabetes status is required annually for all classes of medical certificates.

An applicant with diabetes mellitus - Type II should be counseled by his or her Examiner regarding the significance of the disease and its possible complications.

The applicant should be informed of the potential for hypoglycemic reactions and cautioned to remain under close medical surveillance by his or her treating physician.

The applicant should also be advised that should their medication be changed or the dosage modified, the applicant should not perform airman duties until the applicant and treating physician has concluded that the condition is:

- under control;
- stable;
- presents no risk to aviation safety; and
- consults with the Examiner who issued the certificate, AMCD or RFS.

An applicant who uses insulin for the treatment of his or her diabetes may only be considered for an Authorization for a third-class airman medical certificate.

PROTOCOL FOR DIET CONTROLLED DIABETES MELLITUS AND METABOLIC SYNDROME

(Glucose Intolerance, Impaired Glucose tolerance, Impaired Fasting Glucose, Insulin Resistance, and Pre-Diabetes)

A blood glucose determination is not a routine part of the FAA medical evaluation for any class of medical certificate. However, the examination does include a routine urine test. A medical history or clinical diagnosis of either diabetes mellitus or metabolic syndrome may be considered previously established when the diagnosis has been or clearly could be made because of supporting laboratory findings and/or clinical signs and symptoms. When an applicant with a history of either diabetes or metabolic syndrome is examined for the first time, the Examiner should explain the procedures involved and assist in obtaining prior records and current special testing.

Applicants with a diagnosis of either diabetes mellitus or metabolic syndrome controlled by diet alone are considered eligible for all classes of medical certificates under the medical standards, provided they have no evidence of associated disqualifying cardiovascular, neurological, renal, or ophthalmological disease. Specialized examinations need not be performed unless indicated by history or clinical findings. The Examiner must document these determinations on FAA Form 8500-8.

Protocol for Maximal Graded Exercise Stress Test Requirements

An ECG treadmill stress test should achieve 100% of predicted maximal heart rate unless medically contraindicated or prevented either by symptoms or medications. Studies of less than 85% of maximum predicted heart rate and less than 9 minutes of exercise (6 minutes for age 70 or greater) may serve a basis for denial. Beta blockers and calcium channel blockers (spec. diltiazem and verapamil), or digitalis preparations should be discontinued for 48 hours prior to testing (if not contraindicated) in order to obtain maximum heart rate and only with consent of the treating physician.

The worksheet with blood pressure/pulse recordings at various stages, interpretive report, and actual ECG tracings must be submitted. Tracings must include a rhythm strip, a full 12-lead ECG recorded at rest (supine and standing) and during hyperventilation while standing, one or more times during each stage of exercise, at the end of each stage, at peak exercise, and every minute during recovery for at least 5 minutes or until the tracings return to baseline level. Computer generated, sample-cycle ECG tracings are <u>unacceptable</u> in lieu of the standard tracings. If submitted alone, it may result in deferment until this requirement is met.

In patients with bundle branch blocks, LVH, or diffuse ST/T wave changes at rest, it will be necessary to provide a stress echo or nuclear stress test.

Remember a phone call to either AMCD or RFS may avoid unnecessary deferral.

Reasons for not renewing an AASI:

- The applicant is unable to make at least 85% of maximal heart rate on stress testing or less than 9 minutes (6 minutes if age 70 or greater);

- The applicant develops 1 mm or greater ST segment depression at any time during stress testing. Unless the applicant has additional medical evidence such as a nuclear imaging study or a stress echocardiogram showing the absence of reversible ischemia or wall motion abnormalities reviewed and reported by a qualified cardiologist;

- The nuclear stress testing shows evidence of reversible ischemia, a stress echocardiogram shows exercised induced wall motion abnormalities, or either study demonstrates a negative change from the prior study of the same type;

- The ejection fraction on a nuclear stress test or stress echocardiogram is 40% or less; or a 10% decrease from a prior study; or

- The applicant reports any other disqualifying medical condition or undergoes therapy not previously reported.

Protocol for Graded Exercise Stress Test
Bundle Branch Block Requirements

If the Bundle Branch Block (BBB) has been previously documented and evaluated, no further evaluation is required. A medical certificate should not be issued to any class if the applicant has a new onset of a BBB. A **right** BBB in an otherwise healthy person 30 years of age or younger should not require a CVE. All other individuals who do have a right BBB require a CVE but a radionuclide study should not be required unless the standard exercise stress test cannot be interpreted. A stress echocardiogram may be sufficient in most cases. A **left** BBB in a person of any age should have a CVE and should include a radionuclide perfusion study. **Those individuals who have a negative work-up may be issued the appropriate class of medical certificate. No followup is required.** If any future changes occur, a new current CVE will be required.

If areas of ischemia are noted, a coronary angiogram may be indicated for definitive diagnosis. According to the current literature, approximately 40% of individuals with LBBB will demonstrate a false positive thallium reperfusion defect in the septal area. If significant CAD is diagnosed, refer to Special Issuance guidelines. Some cases may be forwarded to a FAA-selected cardiology consultant specialist for review and recommendation for medical certification.

PROTOCOL FOR HISTORY OF HUMAN IMMUNODEFICIENCY VIRUS (HIV) RELATED CONDITIONS

Persons on antiretroviral medication will be considered only if the medication is approved by the U.S. Food and Drug Administration and is used in accordance with an acceptable drug therapy protocol. Acceptable protocols are cited in *Guidelines for the Use of Antiretroviral Agents in HIV-Infected Adults and Adolescents* developed by the Department of Health and Human Services Panel on Clinical Practices for Treatment of HIV Infection.

Application for special issuance must include reports of examination by a physician knowledgeable in the treatment of HIV-infected persons and a medical history emphasizing symptoms and treatment referable to the immune and neurologic system. In addition, these reports must include a "viral load" determination by polymerase chain reaction (PCR), CD4+ lymphocyte count, a complete blood count, and the results of liver function tests. An assessment of cognitive function (preferably by *Cogscreen* or other test battery acceptable to the Federal Air Surgeon) must be submitted. Additional cognitive function tests may be required as indicated by results of the cognitive tests. At the time of initial application, viral load must not exceed 1,000 copies per milliliter of plasma, and cognitive testing must show no significant deficit(s) that would preclude the safe performance of airman duties.

Followup evaluations of applicants granted certification will include quarterly determinations of viral load by PCR, a CD4+ cell count, and the results of other laboratory and clinical tests deemed appropriate by the treating physician. These will be included in a written status report provided by the treating physician every 6-months. In addition, the results of cognitive function studies will be required at annual intervals for medical clearance or medical certification of ATCS's and first- and second-class applicants. Third-class applicants will be required to submit cognitive function studies every 2 years.

Adverse clinical findings, including significant changes in cognitive test results or an increased viral load exceeding 5,000 copies per milliliter shall constitute a basis for withdrawing medical certification.

Exceptions, if any, will be based on individual consideration by the Federal Air Surgeon.

PROTOCOL FOR EVALUATION OF HYPERTENSION

Initial: The Examiner may issue first-, second-, or third-class medical certificates to otherwise qualified airmen whose hypertension is adequately controlled with acceptable medications without significant adverse effects. In such cases, the Examiner shall:

1. Conduct an evaluation or, at the applicant's option, review the report of a current (within preceding 6 months) cardiovascular evaluation by the applicant's attending physician. This evaluation must include pertinent personal and family medical history, including an assessment of the risk factors for coronary heart disease, a clinical examination including at least three blood pressure readings separated by at least 24-hours each, a resting ECG, and a report of fasting plasma glucose, cholesterol (LDL/HDL), triglycerides, and creatinine levels. A maximal electrocardiographic exercise stress test will be accomplished if it is indicated by history or clinical findings. Specific mention must be made of the medications used, their dosage, and the presence, absence, or history of adverse effects. The initiation of medication or change in dosage is not disqualifying. However, the applicant must not exercise the privileges of the medical certificate for at least 2 weeks. Upon reevaluation, if the blood pressure is controlled without side effects the applicant may resume flying duties. In rare cases where the initial hypertension was severe, additional time may be necessary for normalization of renal and cerebral vascular circulation.

2. Summarize the results of this evaluation in Item 60 of the transmitted application and forward the appropriate documents to the AMCD.

3. Report the results of any additional tests or evaluations that have been accomplished.

4. If appropriate, state in Item 60 on the FAA Form 8500-8 that the applicant's blood pressure is adequately controlled with acceptable medication, there are no known significant adverse effects, and no other cardiovascular, cerebrovascular, or arteriosclerotic disease is evident.

5. Defer certification if the person declines any of the recommended evaluations.

Medications:

- Medications acceptable to the FAA for treatment of hypertension in airmen include all Food and Drug Administration (FDA) approved diuretics, alpha-adrenergic blocking agents, beta-adrenergic blocking agents, calcium channel blocking agents, angiotension converting enzyme (ACE inhibitors) agents, and direct vasodilators.
- NOT acceptable to the FAA:

- o centrally acting agents (such as reserpine, guanethidine, guanadrel, guanabenz, and methyldopa).
  - o A combination of beta-adrenergic blocking agents used with insulin, meglitinides, or sulfonylureas.
- The Examiner must defer issuance of a medical certificate to any applicant whose hypertension has not been evaluated, who uses unacceptable medications, whose medical status is unclear, whose hypertension is uncontrolled, who manifests significant adverse effects of medication, or whose certification has previously been specifically reserved to the FAA.

Followup: Followup evaluations must include a current status report describing at least the medications used and their dosages, the adequacy of blood pressure control, the presence or absence of side effects, the presence or absence of end-organ complications and the results of any appropriate tests or studies. This evaluation can be performed by the Examiner if the Examiner can attest to the accuracy of the above information. Hypertension followups are required annually for first- and second-class medical certificate applicants and at the time of renewal for third-class certificate applicants.

Duration of Certificates: The duration of the certificate will be valid until the time of normal expiration, unless otherwise specified by the FAA.

PROTOCOL FOR EVALUATION OF IMPLANTED PACEMAKER

A 2-month recovery period must elapse after the pacemaker implantation to allow for recovery and stabilization. Submit the following:

1. Copies of hospital/medical records pertaining to the requirement for the pacemaker, make of the generator and leads, model and serial number, admission/discharge summaries, operative report, and all ECG tracings.

2. Evaluation of pacemaker function to include description and documentation of underlying rate and rhythm with the pacer turned "off" or at its lowest setting (pacemaker dependency), programmed pacemaker parameters, surveillance record, and exclusion of myopotential inhibition and pacemaker induced hypotension (pacemaker syndrome), Powerpack data including beginning of life (BOL) and elective replacement indicator/end of life (ERI/EOL).

3. Readable samples of all electronic pacemaker surveillance records post surgery or over the past 6 months, or whichever is longer. It must include a sample strip with pacemaker in free running mode and unless contraindicated, a sample strip with the pacemaker in magnetic mode.

4. An assessment and statement from a physician regarding general physical and cardiac examination to include symptoms or treatment referable to the cardiovascular system; the airman's interim and current cardiac condition, functional capacity, medical history, and medications.

5. A report of current fasting blood sugar and a current blood lipid profile to include: total cholesterol, HDL, LDL, and triglycerides.

6. A current Holter monitor evaluation for at least 24-consecutive hours, to include select representative tracings.

7. A current M-mode, 2-dimensional echocardiogram with Doppler.

8. A current Maximal Graded Exercise Stress Test Requirements

9. It is the responsibility of each applicant to provide the medical information required to determine his/her eligibility for airman medical certification. A medical release form may help in obtaining the necessary information.

All information shall be forwarded in one mailing to:

Medical Appeals Section, AAM-313
Aerospace Medical Certification Division
Federal Aviation Administration
Post Office Box 26080
Oklahoma City OK 73125-9914

Medical Appeals Section, AAM-313
Aerospace Medical Certification Division
Federal Aviation Administration
6700 S MacArthur Blvd., Room B-13
Oklahoma City OK 73169

No consideration can be given for special issuance until all the required data has been received.

The use of the airman's full name and date of birth on all correspondence and reports will aid the agency in locating the proper file.

PROTOCOL FOR MEDICATION CONTROLLED METABOLIC SYNDROME

(Glucose Intolerance, Impaired Glucose tolerance, Impaired Fasting Glucose, Insulin Resistance, and Pre-Diabetes)

This protocol is used for all applicants with Glucose Intolerance, Impaired Glucose tolerance, Impaired Fasting Glucose, Insulin Resistance, and/or Pre-Diabetes treated with oral agents or incretin mimetic medications (exenatide), herein referred to as medication(s).

An applicant with a diagnosis of metabolic syndrome controlled by use of a medication may be considered by the FAA for an Authorization of a Special Issuance of a Medical Certificate (Authorization). Following initiation of medication treatment, a 60-day period must elapse prior to certification to assure stabilization, adequate control, and the absence of side effects or complications from the medication.

The initial Authorization decision is made by the AMCD and may not be made by the Examiner. An Examiner may re-issue a subsequent airman medical certificate under the provisions of the Authorization.

The initial Authorization determination will be made on the basis of a report from the treating physician. There must be sufficient information to rule out diabetes mellitus. For favorable consideration, the report must contain a statement regarding the medication used, dosage, the absence or presence of side effects and clinically significant hypoglycemic episodes, and an indication of satisfactory control of the metabolic syndrome. The results of an A1C hemoglobin determination within the past 30 days must be included. Note must also be made of the presence of cardiovascular, neurological, renal, and/or ophthalmological disease. The presence of one or more of these associated diseases will not be, per se, disqualifying but the disease(s) must be carefully evaluated to determine any added risk to aviation safety.

Re-issuance of a medical certificate under the provisions of an Authorization will also be made on the basis of reports from the treating physician. The contents of the report must contain the same information required for initial issuance and specifically reference the presence or absence of satisfactory control, any change in the dosage or type of medication, and the presence or absence of complications or side effects from the medication. In the event of an adverse change in the applicant's status (development of diabetes mellitus, poor control or complications or side effects from the medication), or the appearance of an associated systemic disease, an Examiner must defer the case with all documentation to the AMCD for consideration.

If, upon further review of the deferred case, AMCD decides that re-issuance is appropriate, the Examiner may again be given the authority to re-issue the medical certificate under the provisions of the Authorization based on data provided by the treating physician, including such information as may be required to assess the status of associated medical condition(s).

At a minimum, followup evaluation by the treating physician of the applicant's metabolic syndrome status is required annually for all classes of medical certificates.

An applicant with metabolic syndrome should be counseled by his or her Examiner regarding the significance of the disease and its possible complications, including the possibility of developing diabetes mellitus.

The applicant should be informed of the potential for hypoglycemic reactions and cautioned to remain under close medical surveillance by his or her treating physician.

The applicant should also be advised that should their medication be changed or the dosage modified, the applicant should not perform airman duties until the applicant and treating physician has concluded that the condition is:

- under control;
- stable;
- presents no risk to aviation safety; and
- consults with the Examiner who issued the certificate, AMCD or RFS.

An applicant who uses insulin for the treatment of his or her metabolic syndrome may only be considered for an Authorization for a third-class airman medical certificate.

PROTOCOL FOR MUSCULOSKELETAL EVALUATION

The Examiner should defer issuance.

An applicant with a history of musculoskeletal conditions must submit the following if consideration for medical certification is desired:

- Current status report

- Functional status report

- Degree of impairment as measured by strength, range of motion, pain

NOTE: If the applicant is otherwise qualified, the FAA may issue a limited certificate. This certificate will permit the applicant to proceed with flight training until ready for a medical flight test. At that time, and at the applicant's request, the FAA (usually the AMCD) will authorize the student pilot to take a medical flight test in conjunction with the regular flight test. The medical flight test and regular private pilot flight test are conducted by an FAA inspector. This affords the student an opportunity to demonstrate the ability to control the aircraft despite the handicap. The FAA inspector prepares a written report and indicates whether there is a safety problem. A medical certificate and statement of demonstrated ability (SODA), without the student limitation, may be provided to the inspector for issuance to the applicant, or the inspector may be required to send the report to the FAA medical officer who authorized the test.

When prostheses are used or additional control devices are installed in an aircraft to assist the amputee, those found qualified by special certification procedures will have their certificates limited to require that the device(s) (and, if necessary, even the specific aircraft) must always be used when exercising the privileges of the airman certificate.

PROTOCOL FOR PEPTIC ULCER

An applicant with a history of an active ulcer within the past 3-months or a bleeding ulcer within the past 6-months must provide evidence that the ulcer is healed if consideration for medical certification is desired.

Evidence of healing must be verified by a report from the attending physician that includes the following information:

- Confirmation that the applicant is free of symptoms

- Radiographic or endoscopic evidence that the ulcer has healed

- The name and dosage medication(s) used for treatment and/or prevention, along with a statement describing side effects or removal

This information should be submitted to the AMCD. Under favorable circumstances, the FAA may issue a certificate with special requirements. For example, an applicant with a history of bleeding ulcer may be required to have the physician submit followup reports every 6-months for 1 year following initial certification.

The prophylactic use of medications including simple antacids, H-2 inhibitors or blockers, proton pump inhibitors, and/or sucralfates may not be disqualifying, if free from side effects.

An applicant with a history of gastric resection for ulcer may be favorably considered if free of sequela.

PROTOCOL FOR RENAL TRANSPLANT

An applicant with a history of renal transplant must submit the following if consideration for medical certification is desired:

1. Hospital admission, operative report and discharge summary

2. Current status report including:

   - The etiology of the primary renal disease

   - History of hypertension or cardiac dysfunction

   - Sequela prior to transplant

   - A comment regarding rejection or graft versus host disease (GVHD)

   - Immunosuppressive therapy and side effects, if any

   - The results of the following laboratory results: CBC, BUN, creatinine, and electrolytes

PROTOCOL FOR
SUBSTANCES OF DEPENDENCE/ABUSE
(DRUGS - ALCOHOL)

The Examiner must defer issuance.

An applicant with a history of substances of dependence/abuse (drugs - alcohol) must submit the following if consideration for medical certification is desired:

- A current status report from a physician certified in addictive disorders and familiar with aviation standards

- A personal statement attesting to the substance and amount, and date last used

- If attended a rehabilitation clinic/center, provide dates and copies of treatment plan

NOTE: The applicant may be required to submit additional information before medical disposition can be rendered.

PROTOCOL FOR THROMBOEMBOLIC DISEASE

An applicant with a history of thromboembolic disease must submit the following if consideration for medical certification is desired:

1. Hospital admission and discharge summary

2. Current status report including:

   - Detailed family history of thromboembolic disease

   - Neoplastic workup, if clinically indicated

   - PT/PTT

   - Protein S & C

   - Leiden Factor V

   - If still anticoagulated, submit all (no less than monthly) INR from time of hospital discharge to present

PROTOCOL FOR CARDIAC VALVE REPLACEMENT

Applicants with tissue and mechanical valve replacement(s) are considered after the following:

- A 6-month recovery period shall elapse after the valve replacement to ensure recovery and stabilization. First- and second-class initial applicants are reviewed by the Federal Air Surgeon's cardiology panel;
- Copies of hospital/medical records pertaining to the valve replacement; include make, model, serial number and size, admission/discharge summaries, operative report, and pathology report;
- If applicable, a current evaluation from the attending physician regarding the use of Coumadin to confirm stability without complications, drug dose history and schedule, and International Normalized Ratio (INR) values (within acceptable range) accomplished at least <u>monthly</u> during the past 6-month period of observation;
- A current report from the treating physician regarding the status of the cardiac valve replacement. This report should address your general cardiovascular condition, any symptoms of valve or heart failure, any related abnormal physical findings, and must substantiate satisfactory recovery and cardiac function without evidence of embolic phenomena, significant arrhythmia, structural abnormality, or ischemic disease.
- A current 24-hour Holter monitor evaluation to include select representative tracings;
- Current M-mode, 2-dimensional echocardiogram with Doppler. Submit the video resulting from this study;
- A current maximal GXT – See GXT Protocol;
- If cardiac catheterization and coronary angiography have been performed, all reports and films must be submitted, if requested, for review by the agency. Copies should be made of all films as a safeguard against loss;.
- Following heart valve replacement, first- and second-class certificate holders shall be followed at 6-month intervals with clinical status reports and at 12-month intervals with a CVE, standard ECG, and Doppler echocardiogram. Holter monitoring and GXT's may be required periodically if indicated clinically. For third-class certificate holders, the above followup testing will be required annually unless otherwise indicated.
- Single, Mechanical and Valvuloplasty - See AASI for Cardiac Valve Replacement;
- Multiple Heart Valve Replacement. Applicants who have received multiple heart valve replacements must be deferred, however, the AMCD may consider certification of all classes of applicants who have undergone a Ross procedure (pulmonic valve transplanted to the aortic position and pulmonic valve replaced by a bioprosthesis).

It is the responsibility of each applicant to provide the medical information required to determine his/her eligibility for airman medical certification. A medical release form may help in obtaining the necessary information.

All information shall be forwarded in <u>one mailing</u> to:

Medical Appeals Section, AAM-313
Aerospace Medical Certification Division
Federal Aviation Administration
Post Office Box 26080
Oklahoma City OK 73125-9914

Medical Appeals Section, AAM-313
Aerospace Medical Certification Division
Federal Aviation Administration
6700 S MacArthur Blvd., Room B-13
Oklahoma City OK 73169

No consideration can be given for Authorization for Special Issuance of a Medical Certificate until all the required data has been received.

Use your full name on any reports or correspondence will aid us in locating your file.

PHARMACEUTICALS

PHARMACEUTICAL MEDICATIONS

As an Examiner you are required to be aware of the regulations and Agency policy and have a responsibility to inform airmen of the potential adverse effects of medications and to counsel airmen regarding their use. There are numerous conditions that require the chronic use of medications that do not compromise aviation safety and, therefore, are permissible. Airmen who develop short-term, self-limited illnesses are best advised to avoid performing aviation duties while medications are used.

Aeromedical decision-making includes an analysis of the underlying disease or condition and treatment. The underlying disease has an equal and often greater influence upon the determination of aeromedical certification. It is unlikely that a source document could be developed and understood by airmen when considering the underlying medical condition(s), drug interactions, medication dosages, and the shear volume of medications that need to be considered. A list may encourage or facilitate an airmen's self-determination of the risks posed by various medical conditions especially when combination therapy is used. A list is subject to misuse if used as the sole factor to determine certification eligibility or compliance with 14 CFR part **61.53**, Prohibition of Operations During Medical Deficiencies. Maintaining a published a list of "acceptable" medications is labor intensive and, in the final analysis, only partially answers the certification question and does not contribute to aviation safety.

Therefore, the list of medications referenced below provides aeromedical guidance about specific medications or classes of pharmaceutical preparations and is applied by using sound aeromedical clinical judgment. This list is not meant to be totally inclusive or comprehensive. No independent interpretation of the FAA's position with respect to a medication included or excluded from the following should be assumed.

ACNE MEDICATIONS
ALLERGY – Antihistamines
ALLERGY – Immunotherapy
ANTACIDS
ANTICOAGULANTS
ANTIDEPRESSANTS
ANTIHYPERTENSIVE
CONTRACEPTIVES AND HORMONE REPLACEMENT THERAPY
DIABETES MELLITUS – Insulin Treated
DIABETES MELLITUS – Type II Medication Controlled (Not Insulin)
GLAUCOMA MEDICATIONS
MALARIA MEDICATION
SEDATIVES

ACNE MEDICATIONS

I. CODE OF FEDERAL REGULATIONS
First-Class Airman Medical Certificate: 67.113(c)
Second-Class Airman Medical Certificate: 67.213(c)
Third-Class Airman Medical Certificate: 67.313(c)

II. MEDICAL HISTORY: For applicants using isotretinoin (Accutane), there is a mandatory 2-week waiting period after starting isotretinoin prior to consideration. **This medication can be associated with vision and psychiatric side effects of aeromedical concern - specifically decreased night vision/ night blindness and depression.** These side-effects can occur even after cessation of isotretinoin. A report must be provided with detailed, specific comment on presence or absence of psychiatric and vision side-effects. The AME must document these findings in Block 60, Comments on History and Findings. Some applicants will have to be deferred. For applicants issued, there must be a "NOT VALID FOR NIGHT FLYING" restriction on the medical certificate. A waiting period and detailed information is required to remove this restriction. The restriction cannot be removed until **all** the requirements are met. See Pharmaceutical Considerations below.

III. AEROMEDICAL DECISION CONSIDERATIONS: See **Item 40,** Skin.
http://www.faa.gov/about/office_org/headquarters_offices/avs/offices/aam/ame/guide/app_process/exam_tech/item40/amd/cutaneous/

IV. PROTOCOL: N/A

V. PHARMACEUTICAL CONSIDERATIONS:

- Use of isotretinoin must be permanently discontinued for at least 2 weeks prior to consideration date (confirmed by the prescribing physician) and;
- Eye evaluation must be done in accordance with specifications in 8500-7 and;
- The airman must provide a signed statement of discontinuation that:
  - Confirms the absence of any visual disturbances and psychiatric symptoms, and
  - Acknowledges requirement to notify the FAA and obtain clearance prior to performing any aviation safety-related duties if use of isotretinoin is resumed

ALLERGY – ANTIHISTAMINES

I. CODE OF FEDERAL REGULATIONS
First-Class Airman Medical Certificate: 67.105(b)(c)
Second-Class Airman Medical Certificate: 67.205(b)(c)
Third-Class Airman Medical Certificate: 67.305(b)(c)

II. MEDICAL HISTORY: Item 18.e., Hay fever or allergy
The applicant should report frequency and duration of symptoms, any incapacitation by the condition, treatment, and side effects. The Examiner should inquire whether the applicant has ever experienced any barotitis ("ear block"), barosinusitis, alternobaric vertigo, or any other symptoms that could interfere with aviation safety.

III. AEROMEDICAL DECISION CONSIDERATIONS: See Item 26, Nose
http://www.faa.gov/about/office_org/headquarters_offices/avs/offices/aam/ame/guide/app_process/exam_tech/item26/amd/
Also, see Aerospace Medical Disposition table and **Item 35**, Lungs and Chest
http://www.faa.gov/about/office_org/headquarters_offices/avs/offices/aam/ame/guide/app_process/exam_tech/item35/amd/

IV. PROTOCOL: See Disease Protocols – Allergies, Severe
http://www.faa.gov/about/office_org/headquarters_offices/avs/offices/aam/ame/guide/dec_cons/disease_prot/antihistamines/

V. PHARMACEUTICAL CONSIDERATIONS:
For hay fever requiring antihistamines:
- The nonsedating antihistamines loratadine, desloratadine, and fexofenadine may be used while flying **if, after an adequate initial "trial period,"** symptoms are controlled without adverse side effects.
- Applicants with seasonal allergies requiring any other antihistamine (oral and/or nasal) may be certified by the examiner **only as follows**:
  - **With the stipulation that they do not exercise the privileges of airman certificate** while taking the medication, AND
  - **Wait after the last dose until** either:
    - At least five maximal dosing intervals* have passed. For example, if the medication is taken every 4-6 hours, wait 30 hours (5x6) after the last dose to fly, or,
    - At least five times the maximum terminal elimination half-life has passed. For example, if the medication half-life* is 6-8 hours, wait 40 hours (5x8) after the last dose to fly.

  * Examiners are encouraged to look up the dosing intervals and half-life.

- For hay fever controlled by **Desensitization**, AME must warn airman to not operate aircraft until **four hours after** each injection.
- Airmen who are exhibiting symptoms, regardless of the treatment used, must not fly.

In all situations, the examiner must notate the evaluation data in Block 60

ALLERGY - IMMUNOTHERAPY

I. CODE OF FEDERAL REGULATIONS
First-Class Airman Medical Certificate: 67.105(b)(c)
Second-Class Airman Medical Certificate: 67.205(b)(c)
Third-Class Airman Medical Certificate: 67.305(b)(c)

II. MEDICAL HISTORY: Item 18.e., Hay fever or allergy.
The applicant should report frequency and duration of symptoms, any incapacitation by the condition, treatment, and side effects. The Examiner should inquire whether the applicant has ever experienced any barotitis ("ear block"), barosinusitis, alternobaric vertigo, or any other symptoms that could interfere with aviation safety.

III. AEROMEDICAL DECISION CONSIDERATIONS: See **Item 26**, Nose, Aerospace Medical Disposition table
http://www.faa.gov/about/office_org/headquarters_offices/avs/offices/aam/ame/guide/app_process/exam_tech/item26/amd/

Also, see Aerospace Medical Disposition table and **Item 35**, Lungs and Chest
http://www.faa.gov/about/office_org/headquarters_offices/avs/offices/aam/ame/guide/app_process/exam_tech/item35/amd/

IV. PROTOCOL - See Disease Protocols – Allergies, Severe
http://www.faa.gov/about/office_org/headquarters_offices/avs/offices/aam/ame/guide/dec_cons/disease_prot/antihistamines/

V. PHARMACEUTICAL CONSIDERATIONS
- For conditions controlled by desensitization, AME must warn the airman to not operate aircraft until **four hours after** each injection.
- Sublingual immunotherapy (SLIT) used for allergic rhinitis is **not** acceptable

ANTACIDS

I. CODE OF FEDERAL REGULATIONS
First-Class Airman Medical Certificate: 67.113(b)(c)
Second-Class Airman Medical Certificate: 67.213(b)(c)
Third-Class Airman Medical Certificate: 67.313(b)(c)

II. MEDICAL HISTORY: Item 18.i.,Stomach, liver, or intestinal trouble.
The applicant should provide history and treatment, pertinent medical records, current status report, and medication. If a surgical procedure was done, the applicant must provide operative and pathology reports.

III. AEROMEDICAL DECISION CONSIDERATIONS: See **Item 38**, Abdomen and Viscera, Aerospace Medical Disposition Table.
http://www.faa.gov/about/office_org/headquarters_offices/avs/offices/aam/ame/guide/app_process/exam_tech/item38/amd/conditions/

IV. PROTOCOL: See Peptic Ulcer
http://www.faa.gov/about/office_org/headquarters_offices/avs/offices/aam/ame/guide/dec_cons/disease_prot/peptic/

V. PHARMACEUTICAL CONSIDERATIONS
The prophylactic use of medications including simple antacids, H-2 inhibitors or blockers, proton pump inhibitors, and/or sucralfates may not be disqualifying, if free from side effects.

ANTICOAGULANTS

I. CODE OF FEDERAL REGULATIONS
First-Class Airman Medical Certificate: 67.113(b)(c)
Second-Class Airman Medical Certificate: 67.213(b)(c)
Third-Class Airman Medical Certificate: 67.313(b)(c)

II. MEDICAL HISTORY: Item 18.g. Heart or vascular trouble.
The applicant should describe the condition to include, dates, symptoms, treatment, and provide medical reports to assist in the certification decision-making process. These reports should include, as indicated by the applicable underlying condition(s) and class applied for: 24-hour Holter monitor, operative reports of any coronary intervention (including the original cardiac catheterization report), stress tests (including worksheets and original tracings or a legible copy). For myocardial perfusion imaging, we require the interpretive report and copies of the actual images in **both** grey-scale and color (in digital format or hard copy.) Per Part 67, for all classes of medical certificates, there is cause for denial if there is an established medical history or clinical diagnosis of myocardial infarction, angina pectoris, cardiac valve replacement, permanent cardiac pacemaker implantation, heart replacement, or coronary heart disease that has required treatment (or if untreated, that has been symptomatic or clinically significant).

III. AEROMEDICAL DECISION CONSIDERATIONS: See Item 36, Heart,
Aerospace Medical Disposition table
http://www.faa.gov/about/office_org/headquarters_offices/avs/offices/aam/ame/guide/app_process/exam_tech/item36/amd/

IV. PROTOCOL: As per the specific underlying condition(s), see
http://www.faa.gov/about/office_org/headquarters_offices/avs/offices/aam/ame/guide/dec_cons/disease_prot/

V. PHARMACEUTICAL CONSIDERATIONS
For applicants using warfarin (Coumadin), the status report from the treating physician should address drug dose history and schedule, comment regarding side effects, and include a minimum of monthly International Normalized Ratio (INR) results for the immediate prior 6 months.

ANTIDEPRESSANTS

I. CODE OF FEDERAL REGULATIONS
    First-Class Airman Medical Certificate: 67.107
    Second-Class Airman Medical Certificate: 67.207
    Third-Class Airman Medical Certificate: 67.307

II. MEDICAL HISTORY: **Item 18.m.,** Mental disorders of any sort; depression, anxiety, etc.

An affirmative answer to Item 18.m. requires investigation through supplemental history taking. Dispositions will vary according to the details obtained. An applicant with an established history of a personality disorder that is severe enough to have repeatedly manifested itself by overt acts, a psychosis disorder, or a bipolar disorder must be denied or deferred by the Examiner.

III. AEROMEDICAL DECISION CONSIDERATIONS: See **Item 47.**, Psychiatric, Aerospace Medical Disposition table.

IV. PROTOCOL: See Aerospace Medical Dispositions, **Item 47**., Psychiatric Conditions

V. PHARMACEUTICAL CONSIDERATIONS
The use of a psychotropic drug is disqualifying for aeromedical certification purposes – this includes all antidepressant drugs, including selective serotonin reuptake inhibitors (SSRIs). However, the FAA has determined that airmen requesting first, second, or third class medical certificates while being treated with one of four specific SSRIs may be considered (see Item 47., Psychiatric Conditions – Use of Antidepressant Medications). The Autorization decision is made on a case by case basis. **The Examiner may not issue.**

ANTIHYPERTENSIVE

I. CODE OF FEDERAL REGULATIONS
First-Class Airman Medical Certificate: 67.113(b)(c)
Second-Class Airman Medical Certificate: 67.213(b)(c)
Third-Class Airman Medical Certificate: 67.313(b)(c)

II. MEDICAL HISTORY: Item 18.h., High or low blood pressure.
The applicant should provide history and treatment, type of medication, purpose, and duration of use. Issuance of a medical certificate is dependant on current blood pressure levels and whether the applicant is taking anti-hypertensive medication. The Examiner should also determine if the applicant has a history of complications, adverse reactions to therapy, hospitalization, etc.

III. AEROMEDICAL DECISION CONSIDERATIONS: See Item 36, Heart – Hypertension
http://www.faa.gov/about/office_org/headquarters_offices/avs/offices/aam/ame/guide/app_process/exam_tech/item36/amd/hypertension/
Also see **Item 55**, Blood Pressure
http://www.faa.gov/about/office_org/headquarters_offices/avs/offices/aam/ame/guide/app_process/exam_tech/item55/amd/

IV. PROTOCOL: See Hypertension Protocol
http://www.faa.gov/about/office_org/headquarters_offices/avs/offices/aam/ame/guide/dec_cons/disease_prot/hypertension/

V. PHARMACEUTICAL CONSIDERATIONS
- Medications acceptable to the FAA for treatment of hypertension in airmen include all Food and Drug Administration (FDA) approved diuretics, alpha-adrenergic blocking agents, beta-adrenergic blocking agents, calcium channel blocking agents, angiotension converting enzyme (ACE inhibitors) agents, and direct vasodilators.

- NOT acceptable to the FAA:
  o Centrally acting agents (such as reserpine, guanethidine, guanadrel, guanabenz, and methyldopa).
  o A combination of beta-adrenergic blocking agents used with insulin, meglitinides, or sulfonylureas.
- The Examiner must defer issuance of a medical certificate to any applicant whose hypertension has not been evaluated, who uses unacceptable medications, whose medical status is unclear, whose hypertension is uncontrolled, who manifests significant adverse effects of medication, or whose certification has previously been specifically reserved to the FAA.

CONTRACEPTIVES AND
HORMONE REPLACEMENT THERAPY

I. CODE OF FEDERAL REGULATIONS
    First-Class Airman Medical Certificate: 67.113(b)(c)
    Second-Class Airman Medical Certificate: 67.213(b)(c)
    Third-Class Airman Medical Certificate: 67.313(b)(c)

II. MEDICAL HISTORY: Use of Oral or Repository Contraceptives or Hormonal Replacement Therapy are not disqualifying for medical certification. If the applicant is experiencing no adverse symptoms or reactions to hormones and is otherwise qualified, the Examiner may issue the desired certificate.

III. AEROMEDICAL DECISION CONSIDERATIONS: See Medical History above and **Item 41., G-U-System,** Gender Identity Disorder

IV. PROTOCOL: N/A

V. PHARMACEUTICAL CONSIDERATIONS: See Medical History above.

DIABETES MELLITUS - INSULIN TREATED

I. CODE OF FEDERAL REGULATIONS
First-Class Airman Medical Certificate: 67.113(a)(b)(c)
Second-Class Airman Medical Certificate: 67.213(a)(b)(c)
Third-Class Airman Medical Certificate: 67.313(a)(b)(c)

II. MEDICAL HISTORY: Item 18.k., Diabetes.
The applicant should describe the condition to include, symptoms and treatment. Comment on the presence or absence of hyperglycemic and/or hypoglycemic episodes. A medical history or clinical diagnosis of diabetes mellitus requiring insulin or other hypoglycemic drugs for control are disqualifying. The Examiner can help expedite the FAA review by assisting the applicant in gathering medical records and submitting a current specialty report.

III. AEROMEDICAL DECISION CONSIDERATIONS: See Item 48,
General Systemic Aerospace Medical Disposition table.
http://www.faa.gov/about/office_org/headquarters_offices/avs/offices/aam/ame/guide/app_process/exam_tech/item48/amd/diabetes/
The FAA has established a policy that permits the special issuance medical certification of insulin treated applicants for **third class medical certification only**. Consideration will be given only to those individuals who have been clinically stable on their current treatment regimen for a period of 6-months or more.

IV. PROTOCOL: See Insulin-Treated Diabetes Mellitus - Type I or Type II, Protocol
http://www.faa.gov/about/office_org/headquarters_offices/avs/offices/aam/ame/guide/dec_cons/disease_prot/diabetes_insulin/

V. PHARMACEUTICAL CONSIDERATIONS
- Insulin pumps are an acceptable form of treatment.
- Combination of insulin with beta-bockers is not permitted

Combination of insulin with other anti-diabetes medication (s): not all combinations of DM medications are allowed by the FAA, even if each medication within the combination is acceptable as monotherapy. Contact Regional Flight Surgeon's office or AMCD.

DIABETES MELLITUS – TYPE II
MEDICATION CONTROLLED (NOT INSULIN)

I. CODE OF FEDERAL REGULATIONS
First-Class Airman Medical Certificate: 67.113 (a)(b)(c)
Second-Class Airman Medical Certificate: 67.213(a)(b)(c)
Third-Class Airman Medical Certificate: 67.313(a)(b)(c)

II. MEDICAL HISTORY: Item 18.k. Diabetes.
The applicant should describe the condition to include symptoms and treatment. Comment on the presence or absence of hyperglycemic and/or hypoglycemic episodes. A medical history or clinical diagnosis of diabetes mellitus requiring insulin or other hypoglycemic drugs for control is disqualifying. The Examiner can help expedite the FAA review by assisting the applicant in gathering medical records and submitting a current specialty report.

III. AEROMEDICAL DECISION CONSIDERATIONS: See Item 48, Diabetes
http://www.faa.gov/about/office_org/headquarters_offices/avs/offices/aam/ame/guide/app_process/exam_tech/item48/amd/diabetes/

IV. DISEASE PROTOCOL: See Diabetes Mellitus-Type II, Medication Controlled
http://www.faa.gov/about/office_org/headquarters_offices/avs/offices/aam/ame/guide/dec_cons/disease_prot/diabetes_med/

V. PHARMACEUTICAL CONSIDERATIONS
   a. Combination of DM medications with antihypertensives:

- Disqualifying Combinations. Certification of airmen using meglitinides or sulfonylureas, along with beta-blockers is not permitted. Commonly used meglitinides include repaglinide (Prandin) and nateglinide (Starlix). Commonly used sulfonylureas include: acetohexamide (Dymelor); chloropropamide (Diabinese); tolazamide (Tolinase); tolbutamide (Orinase); glimepiride (Amaryl); glipizide (Glucotrol, Glucotrol XL); glyburide (DiaBeta, Micronase, Glynase); glyburide plus metformin (Glucovance); glipizide plus metformin (Metaglip).

- Allowable Combinations. Certification of airmen using the combination of a beta-blocker with the following diabetes medications is permitted: alpha-glucosidase inhibitors [acarbose (Precose), miglitol (Glyset)]; biguanides [metformin (Glucophage)]; thiazolidinediones [pioglitazone (Actos)]; DDP-4 inhibitors [sitagliptin (Januvia)]; and incretin mimetics [exenatide (Byetta)].

GLAUCOMA MEDICATIONS

I. CODE OF FEDERAL REGULATIONS
First-Class Airman Medical Certificate: 67.113(b)(c)
Second-Class Airman Medical Certificate: 67.213 (b)(c)
Third-Class Airman Medical Certificate: 67.313(b)(c)

II. MEDICAL HISTORY: **Item 18.,d,** Medical History, Eye or vision trouble except glasses.
The applicant should provide history and treatment, pertinent medical records, current status report, and medication and dosage.

III. AEROMEDICAL DECISION CONSIDERATIONS: See **Item 32**,
Ophthalmoscopic
http://www.faa.gov/about/office_org/headquarters_offices/avs/offices/aam/ame/g uide/app_process/exam_tech/item32/amd/

IV. PROTOCOL: N/A

V. PHARMACEUTICAL CONSIDERATIONS

A few applicants have been certified following their demonstration of adequate control with oral medication. Neither miotics nor mydriatics are necessarily medically disqualifying. However, miotics such as pilocarpine cause pupillary constriction and could conceivably interfere with night vision.

Although the FAA no longer routinely prohibits pilots who use such medications from flying at night, it may be worthwhile for the Examiner to discuss this aspect of the use of miotics with applicants. If considerable disturbance in night vision is documented, the FAA may limit the medical certificate: NOT VALID FOR NIGHT FLYING.

MALARIA MEDICATIONS

I. CODE OF FEDERAL REGULATIONS
First-Class Airman Medical Certificate: 67.113(c)
Second-Class Airman Medical Certificate: 67.213(c)
Third-Class Airman Medical Certificate: 67.313(c)

II. MEDICAL HISTORY: Mefloquine (Lariam) is associated with adverse neuropsychiatric side-effects, even weeks after the drug is discontinued. This medication is absolutely disqualifying for pilots. Because of the association with adverse neuropsychiatric side-effects, even weeks after discontinuation, a pilot who elects to use mefloquine for malaria prophylaxis or who contracts malaria and is treated with mefloquine will be disqualified for pilot duties for the duration of use of mefloquine and for 4 weeks after the last dose. In this instance, the pilot **must contact the FAA** or his/her Aviation Medical Examiner prior to returning to flight duties after use.

III. AEROMEDICAL DECISION CONSIDERATIONS: See Medical History above.

IV. PROTOCOL: N/A

V. PHARMACEUTICAL CONSIDERATIONS: See Medical History above.

SEDATIVES

I. CODE OF FEDERAL REGULATIONS
First-Class Airman Medical Certificate: 67.107
Second-Class Airman Medical Certificate: 67.207
Third-Class Airman Medical Certificate: 67.307

II. MEDICAL HISTORY and CONVICTIONS OR ADMINISTRATIVE ACTIONS.
Medical History: Item **18.n.**, Substance Dependence; or failed a drug test ever; or substance abuse or use of illegal substance in the last 2 years.

"Substance" includes alcohol and other drugs (e.g., PCP, sedatives and hypnotics, anxiolytics, marijuana, cocaine, opioids, amphetamines, hallucinogens, and other psychoactive drugs or chemicals). For a "yes" answer to Item 18.n., the Examiner should obtain a detailed description of the history. A history of substance dependence or abuse is disqualifying. The Examiner must defer issuance of a certificate if there is doubt concerning an applicant's substance use.

Convictions or Administrative Actions: Item **18.v.**, Conviction and/or Administrative Action History

The events to be reported are specifically identified in Item 18.v. of FAA Form 8500-8. If "yes" is checked, the applicant must describe the conviction(s) and/or administrative action(s) in the EXPLANATIONS box. The description must include:
- The alcohol or drug offense for which the applicant was convicted or the type of administrative action involved (e.g., attendance at an educational or rehabilitation program in lieu of conviction; license denial, suspension, cancellation, or revocation for refusal to be tested; educational safe driving program for multiple speeding convictions; etc.);
- The name of the state or other jurisdiction involved; and
- The date of the conviction and/or administrative action

If there have been no new convictions or administrative actions since the last application, the applicant may enter "PREVIOUSLY REPORTED, NO CHANGE." Convictions and/or administrative actions affecting driving privileges may raise questions about the applicant's fitness for certification and may be cause for disqualification.

A single driving while intoxicated (DWI) conviction or administrative action usually is not cause for denial if there are no other instances or indications of substance dependence or abuse. The Examiner should inquire regarding the applicant's alcohol use history, the circumstances surrounding the incident, and document those findings in **Item 60.**

NOTE: The Examiner should advise the applicant that the reporting of alcohol or drug offenses (i.e., motor vehicle violation) on the history part of the medical application does not relieve the airman of responsibility to report each motor vehicle action to the FAA within 60 days of the occurrence to the Civil Aviation Security Division, AAC-700; P.O. Box 25810; Oklahoma City, OK 73125-0810.

III. AEROMEDICAL DECISION CONSIDERATIONS: See Item 47., Psychiatric, Aerospace Medical Disposition table.

IV. PROTOCOL: See Substances of Dependence/Abuse Protocol

V. PHARMACEUTICAL CONSIDERATIONS

   A. Aerospace Medical Dispositions, Item 47. Psychiatric Conditions

SPECIAL ISSUANCES

AASIs for ALL CLASSES
AASIs for THIRD-CLASS

AASI COVERSHEET

LAST UPDATE: December 14, 2012

Authorization for Special Issuance of a Medical Certificate and AME Assisted Special Issuance (AASI)

A. Special Issuance.

At his discretion, the Federal Air Surgeon may grant an Authorization for Special Issuance of a Medical Certificate (Authorization), with a specified validity period, to an applicant who does not meet the established medical standards. The applicant must demonstrate to the satisfaction of the Federal Air Surgeon that the duties authorized by the class of medical certificate applied for can be performed without endangering public safety for the validity period of the Authorization. The Federal Air Surgeon may authorize a special medical flight test, practical test, or medical evaluation for this purpose. An airman medical certificate issued under the provisions of an Authorization expires no later than the Authorization expiration date or upon its withdrawal. An airman must again show to the satisfaction of the Federal Air Surgeon that the duties authorized by the class of medical certificate applied for can be performed without endangering public safety in order to obtain a new airman medical certificate/Authorization under Title 14 of the Code of Federal Regulations (14 CFR) §67.401.

See Title 14 of the Code of Federal Regulations (14 CFR) §67.401.

B. AME Assisted Special Issuance (AASI).

AME Assisted Special Issuance (AASI) is a process that provides Examiners the ability to re-issue an airman medical certificate under the provisions of an Authorization to an applicant who has a medical condition that is disqualifying under 14 CFR Part 67.

An FAA physician provides the initial certification decision and grants the Authorization in accordance with 14 CFR § 67.401. The Authorization letter is accompanied by attachments that specify the information that treating physician(s) must provide for the re-issuance determination. Examiners may re-issue an airman medical certificate under the provisions of an Authorization, if the applicant provides the requisite medical information required for determination. Examiners may not issue initial Authorizations. An Examiner's decision or determination is subject to review by the FAA

AME Assisted Special Issuance (AASI)

The following pages of the Guide for Aviation Medical Examiners introduce the AME Assisted Special Issuance (AASI) process.

If this is a first-time issuance for a disqualifying disease/condition, and the applicant has all of the requisite medical information necessary for a determination, the Examiner must defer, and submit all of the documentation to the AMCD or your RFS.

The Guide refers to a number of selected medical conditions that are initially disqualifying and must be deferred to the AMCD or RFS. Following the granting of an Authorization for Special Issuance of a Medical Certificate (Authorization) by the AMCD or RFS. Each AASI has their own specialized clinical criteria, by which an Examiner may reissue a medical certificate to an applicant with a medical history of an initially disqualifying condition, if otherwise qualified.

ARTHRITIS and/ or PSORIASIS

ASTHMA

ATRIAL FIBRILLATION

BLADDER CANCER

BREAST CANCER

CHRONIC LYMPHOCYTIC LEUKEMIA

CHRONIC OBSTRUCTIVE PULMONARY DISEASE

COLITIS
(Ulcerative or Crohn's Disease)

COLON CANCER

DEEP VEIN THROMBOSIS/ PULMONARY EMBOLISM
Warfarin (Coumadin) Therapy

DIABETES MELLITUS – TYPE II
Medication Controlled (Not Insulin)

GLAUCOMA

HEPATITIS C

HYERTHYROIDISM

HYPOTHYROIDISM

LYMPHOMA and HODGKIN'S DISEASE

MELANOMA

METABOLIC SYNDROME
(Glucose Intolerance, Impaired Glucose Tolerance, Impaired Fasting Glucose, Insulin Resistance and Pre-Diabetes)

MIGRAINE HEADACHES

MITRAL and AORTIC INSUFFICIENCY

PAROXYSMAL ATRIAL TACHYCARDIA

PROSTATE CANCER

RENAL CALCULI

RENAL CARCINOMA

SLEEP APNEA

TESTICULAR CANCER

AASI FOR ARTHRITIS AND/ OR PSORIASIS

AME Assisted Special Issuance (AASI) is a process that provides Examiners the ability to re-issue an airman medical certificate under the provisions of an Authorization for Special Issuance of a Medical Certificate (Authorization) to an applicant who has a medical condition that is disqualifying under Title 14 of the Code of Federal Regulations (14 CFR) part 67.

An FAA physician provides the initial certification decision and grants the Authorization in accordance with 14 CFR § 67.401. The Authorization letter is accompanied by attachments which specify the information that treating physician(s) must provide for the re-issuance determination. If this is a first-time issuance of an Authorization for the above disease/condition, and the applicant has all of the requisite medical information necessary for a determination, the Examiner must defer and submit all of the documentation to the AMCD or RFS for the initial determination.

Examiners may re-issue an airman medical certificate under the provisions of an Authorization, if the applicant provides the following:

- An Authorization granted by the FAA;
- The type of arthritis or psoriasis;
- A general assessment of the condition and its effect on daily activities;
- The name and dosage of medication(s) used for treatment and/or prevention with comment regarding side effects; and
- For arthritis - comments regarding range of motion of neck, upper and lower extremities, hands, etc.

The Examiner must defer to the AMCD or Region if:

- The applicant has developed any associated systemic manifestations;
- For arthritis - new joints have become involved;
- The applicant required change in medication used for control of the disease; or
- The applicant is on greater than 20mg of prednisone-equivalent daily

AASI FOR ASTHMA

Note: If the applicant has mild symptoms that are infrequent, have not required hospitalization, or use of steroid medication, and no symptoms in flight, the Examiner may issue an airman medical certificate. See Item 35., Lungs and Chest Aerospace Medical Disposition.

If the applicant does not meet the above criteria, the Examiner must follow the AASI process.

AME Assisted Special Issuance (AASI) is a process that provides Examiners the ability to re-issue an airman medical certificate under the provisions of an Authorization for Special Issuance of a Medical Certificate (Authorization) to an applicant who has a medical condition that is disqualifying under Title 14 of the Code of Federal Regulations (14 CFR) part 67.

An FAA physician provides the initial certification decision and grants the Authorization in accordance with 14 CFR § 67.401. The Authorization letter is accompanied by attachments that specify the information that treating physician(s) must provide for the re-issuance determination. If this is a first time issuance of an Authorization for the above disease/condition, and the applicant has all of the requisite medical information necessary for a determination, the Examiner must defer and submit all of the documentation to the AMCD or RFS for the initial determination.

Examiners may re-issue an airman medical certificate under the provisions of an Authorization, if the applicant provides the following:

- An Authorization granted by the FAA;
- The applicant's current medical status that addresses frequency of attacks and whether the attacks have resulted in emergency room visits or hospitalizations;
- The Examiner should caution the applicant to cease flying with any exacerbation as warned in § 61.53;
- The name and dosage of medication(s) used for treatment and/or prevention with comment regarding side effects; and
- Results of pulmonary function testing, if deemed necessary, performed within the last 90 days

The Examiner must defer to the AMCD or Region if:

- The symptoms worsen;
- There has been an increase in frequency of emergency room, hospital, or outpatient visits;
- The FEV1 is less than 70% predicted value;
- The applicant requires 3 or more medications for stabilization; or
- The applicant is using steroids in dosages equivalent to more than 20mg of Prednisone per day.

AASI FOR ATRIAL FIBRILLATION

AME Assisted Special Issuance (AASI) is a process that provides Examiners the ability to re-issue an airman medical certificate under the provisions of an Authorization for Special Issuance of a Medical Certificate (Authorization) to an applicant who has a medical condition that is disqualifying under Title 14 of the Code of Federal Regulations (14 CFR) part 67.

An FAA physician provides the initial certification decision and grants the Authorization in accordance with 14 CFR § 67.401. The Authorization letter is accompanied by attachments that specify the information that treating physician(s) must provide for the re-issuance determination. If this is a first time issuance of an Authorization for the above disease/condition, and the applicant has all the requisite medical information necessary for a determination, the Examiner must defer and submit all of the documentation to the AMCD or RFS for the initial determination.

Examiners may re-issue an airman medical certificate under the provisions of an Authorization, if the applicant provides the following:

- An Authorization granted by the FAA;
- A summary of the applicant's medical condition since the last FAA medical examination, including a statement regarding any further episodes of atrial fibrillation;
- The name and dosage of medication(s) used for treatment and/or prevention with comment regarding side effects;
- A report of a current 24-hour Holter Monitor performed within the last 90 days;
- A minimum of monthly International Normalized Ratio (INR) results for the immediate prior 6 months, for airmen being treated with warfarin (Coumadin).

The Examiner must defer to the AMCD or Region if:

- Holter Monitor demonstrates: HR >120 BPM or Pauses >3 seconds;
- More than 20% of INR values are <2.0 or >3.0; or
- The applicant develops emboli, thrombosis, bleeding that required medical intervention, or any other cardiac condition previously not diagnosed or reported.

AASI FOR BLADDER CANCER

AME Assisted Special Issuance (AASI) is a process that provides Examiners the ability to re-issue an airman medical certificate under the provisions of an Authorization for Special Issuance of a Medical Certificate (Authorization) to an applicant who has a medical condition that is disqualifying under Title 14 of the Code of Federal Regulations (14 CFR) part 67.

An FAA physician provides the initial certification decision and grants the Authorization in accordance with 14 CFR § 67.401. The Authorization letter is accompanied by attachments that specify the information that treating physician(s) must provide for the re-issuance determination. If this is a first time issuance of an Authorization for the above disease/condition, and the applicant has all of the requisite medical information necessary for a determination, the Examiner must defer and submit all of the documentation to the AMCD or RFS for the initial determination.

Examiners may re-issue an airman medical certificate under the provisions of an Authorization, if the applicant provides the following:

- An Authorization granted by the FAA; and
- A current status report performed within 90 days that must include all the required followup items and studies as listed in the Authorization letter and that confirms absence of recurrent disease

The Examiner must defer to the AMCD or Region if:

- There has been any recurrence of the cancer; or
- Any new treatment is initiated

AASI FOR BREAST CANCER

AME Assisted Special Issuance (AASI) is a process that provides Examiners the ability to re-issue an airman medical certificate under the provisions of an Authorization for Special Issuance of a Medical Certificate (Authorization) to an applicant who has a medical condition that is disqualifying under Title 14 of the Code of Federal Regulations (14 CFR) part 67.

An FAA physician provides the initial certification decision and grants the Authorization in accordance with 14 CFR § 67.401. The Authorization letter is accompanied by attachments that specify the information that treating physician(s) must provide for the re-issuance determination. If this is a first time issuance of an Authorization for the above disease/condition, and the applicant has all of the requisite medical information necessary for a determination, the Examiner must defer and submit all of the documentation to the AMCD or RFS for the initial determination.

Examiners may re-issue an airman medical certificate under the provisions of an Authorization, if the applicant provides the following:

- An Authorization granted by the FAA; and
- A current status report performed within the last 90 days that must include all the required followup items and studies as listed in the Authorization letter and that confirms absence of recurrent disease.

The Examiner must defer to the AMCD or Region if:

- There has been any recurrence of the cancer; or
- Any new treatment is initiated.

AASI FOR CHRONIC LYMPHOCYTIC LEUKEMIA

AME Assisted Special Issuance (AASI) is a process that provides Examiners the ability to re-issue an airman medical certificate under the provisions of an Authorization for Special Issuance of a Medical Certificate (Authorization) to an applicant who has a medical condition that is disqualifying under Title 14 of the Code of Federal Regulations (14 CFR) part 67.

An FAA physician provides the initial certification decision and grants the Authorization in accordance with 14 CFR § 67.401. The Authorization letter is accompanied by attachments that specify the information that treating physician(s) must provide for the re-issuance determination. If this is a first time issuance of an Authorization for the above disease/condition, and the applicant has all of the requisite medical information necessary for a determination, the Examiner must defer and submit all of the documentation to the AMCD or RFS for the initial determination.

Examiners may re-issue an airman medical certificate under the provisions of an Authorization, if the applicant provides the following:

- An Authorization granted by the FAA;
- A clinical followup report from the treating physician that includes an update of the condition of the applicant since the last examination; and
- The results of any applicable laboratory results, including a complete blood count performed within the last 90 days.

The Examiner must defer to the AMCD or Region if:

- The condition currently requires treatment with a chemotherapeutic agent; or
- The white blood cell count has risen above 80,000; or
- Any new treatment is initiated

AASI FOR
CHRONIC OBSTRUCTIVE PULMONARY DISEASE

AME Assisted Special Issuance (AASI) is a process that provides Examiners the ability to re-issue an airman medical certificate under the provisions of an Authorization for Special Issuance of a Medical Certificate (Authorization) to an applicant who has a medical condition that is disqualifying under Title 14 of the Code of Federal Regulations (14 CFR) part 67.

An FAA physician provides the initial certification decision and grants the Authorization in accordance with 14 CFR § 67.401. The Authorization letter is accompanied by attachments that specify the information that treating physician(s) must provide for the re-issuance determination. If this is a first time issuance of an Authorization for the above disease/condition, and the applicant has all of the requisite medical information necessary for a determination, the Examiner must defer and submit all of the documentation to the AMCD or RFS for the initial determination.

Examiners may re-issue an airman medical certificate under the provisions of an Authorization, if the applicant provides the following:

- An Authorization granted by the FAA;
- A statement regarding symptomatology of the condition;
- A statement addressing any associated illnesses, such as heart failure;
- The name and dosage of medication(s) used for treatment and/or prevention with comment regarding side effects; and
- A pulmonary specialist evaluation that includes the results of a current pulmonary function test, performed within the last 90 days

The Examiner must defer to the AMCD or Region if:

- The FEV1 or FEV1/FVC is less than 70%;
- The applicant has been placed on a steroid dose equivalent to greater than 20mg of Prednisone per day; or
- The applicant has developed an associated cardiac condition.

AASI FOR COLITIS
(ULCERATIVE OR CROHN'S DISEASE)

AME Assisted Special Issuance (AASI) is a process that provides Examiners the ability to re-issue an airman medical certificate under the provisions of an Authorization for Special Issuance of a Medical Certificate (Authorization) to an applicant who has a medical condition that is disqualifying under Title 14 of the Code of Federal Regulations (14 CFR) part 67.

An FAA physician provides the initial certification decision and grants the Authorization in accordance with 14 CFR § 67.401. The Authorization letter is accompanied by attachments that specify the information that treating physician(s) must provide for the re-issuance determination. If this is a first time issuance of an Authorization for the above disease/condition, and the applicant has all of the requisite medical information necessary for a determination, the Examiner must defer and submit all of the documentation to the AMCD or RFS for the initial determination.

Examiners may re-issue an airman medical certificate under the provisions of an Authorization, if the applicant provides the following:

- An Authorization granted by the FAA;
- A statement regarding the extent of disease;
- A statement regarding the frequency of exacerbation (the applicant should cease flying with any exacerbation as warned in § 61.53); and
- The name and dosage of medication(s) used for treatment and/or prevention with comment regarding side effects.

The Examiner must defer to the AMCD or Region if:

- There is a current exacerbation of the illness;
- The applicant is taking medications such as Lomotil, steroid doses equivalent to more than 20mg of Prednisone per day, antispasmodics, and anticholinergics; or
- The pattern of exacerbations are increasing in frequency or severity; or applicant underwent surgical intervention.

AASI FOR COLON/COLORECTAL CANCER

AME Assisted Special Issuance (AASI) is a process that provides Examiners the ability to re-issue an airman medical certificate under the provisions of an Authorization for Special Issuance of a Medical Certificate (Authorization) to an applicant who has a medical condition that is disqualifying under Title 14 of the Code of Federal Regulations (14 CFR) part 67.

An FAA physician provides the initial certification decision and grants the Authorization in accordance with 14 CFR § 67.401. The Authorization letter is accompanied by attachments that specify the information that treating physician(s) must provide for the re-issuance determination. If this is a first time issuance of an Authorization for the above disease/condition, and the applicant has all of the requisite medical information necessary for a determination, the Examiner must defer and submit all of the documentation to the AMCD or RFS for the initial determination.

Examiners may re-issue an airman medical certificate under the provisions of an Authorization, if the applicant provides the following:

- An Authorization granted by the FAA; and
- An update of the status of the malignancy since the last FAA medical examination, to include the results of a current (performed within the last 90 days) carcinoembryonic antigen (CEA), if a baseline value is available

The Examiner must defer to the AMCD or Region if:

- There has been any progression of the disease or an increase in CEA
- Any new treatment is initiated

AASI FOR DIABETES MELLITUS - TYPE II MEDICATION CONTROLLED (NOT INSULIN)

AME Assisted Special Issuance (AASI) is a process that provides Examiners the ability to re-issue an airman medical certificate under the provisions of an Authorization for Special Issuance of a Medical Certificate (Authorization) to an applicant who has a medical condition that is disqualifying under Title 14 of the Code of Federal Regulations (14 CFR) part 67.

An FAA physician provides the initial certification decision and grants the Authorization in accordance with 14 CFR § 67.401. The Authorization letter is accompanied by attachments that specify the information that treating physician(s) must provide for the re-issuance determination. If this is a first time issuance of an Authorization for the above disease/condition, and the applicant has provided all of the requisite medical information necessary for a determination, the Examiner must defer and submit all of the documentation to the AMCD or RFS for the initial determination.

Examiners may re-issue an airman medical certificate under the provisions of an Authorization, if the applicant provides the following:

- An Authorization granted by the FAA;
- A current status report from the physician treating the airman's diabetes, including:
    - A statement attesting that the airman is maintaining his or her diabetic diet;
    - A statement regarding any diabetic symptomatology; including any history of hypoglycemic events and any cardiovascular, renal, neurologic, or ophthalmologic complications; and
    - The results of a current HgA1c level performed within last 30 days.

The Examiner must defer to the AMCD or Region if:

- The applicant has been placed on insulin;
- The HgA1c level is greater than 9.0 mg%
- Any hypoglycemic event
- The applicant has developed evidence of any of the following:
    - Cardiovascular disease,
    - Neurologic disease, including any change in degree of peripheral neuropathy,
    - Ophthalmologic disease,
    - Renal disease (including a Creatinine over 2.0)
- The airman has been placed on any amlynomimetics, such as pramlintide (Symlin)
- There is a change in oral hypoglycemic medication
- The airman has been placed on beta-blockers AND his/her oral diabetes medications include any sulfonlyurea and/or any meglitinide. **Commonly used meglitinides include repaglinide (Prandin) and nateglinide (Starlix). Commonly used sulfonylureas include: acetohexamide (Dymelor); chloropropamide (Diabinese); tolazamide (Tolinase); tolbutamide (Orinase); glimepiride (Amaryl); glipizide (Glucotrol, Glucotrol XL); glyburide (DiaBeta, Micronase, Glynase); glyburide plus metformin (Glucovance); glipizide plus metformin (Metaglip).**
- Any new treatment is initiated

AASI FOR GLAUCOMA

AME Assisted Special Issuance (AASI) is a process that provides Examiners the ability to re-issue an airman medical certificate under the provisions of an Authorization for Special Issuance of a Medical Certificate (Authorization) to an applicant who has a medical condition that is disqualifying under Title 14 of the Code of Federal Regulations (14 CFR) part 67.

An FAA physician provides the initial certification decision and grants the Authorization in accordance with 14 CFR § 67.401. The Authorization letter is accompanied by attachments that specify the information that treating physician(s) must provide for the re-issuance determination. If this is a first time issuance of an Authorization for the above disease/condition, and the applicant has all of the requisite medical information necessary for a determination, the Examiner must defer and submit all of the documentation to the AMCD or RFS for the initial determination.

Examiners may re-issue an airman medical certificate under the provisions of an Authorization, if the applicant provides the following:

- An Authorization granted by the FAA;
- Certification only granted for open-angle-glaucoma and ocular hypertension;
- The FAA Form 8500-14, Glaucoma Eye Evaluation Form is filled out by the treating eye specialist; and
- A set of visual fields measurements is provided.

The Examiner must defer to the AMCD or Region if:

- The FAA Form 8500-14 Glaucoma Eye Evaluation Form demonstrates visual acuity incompatible with the medical standards; or
- There is a change in visual fields or adverse change in ocular pressure.

AASI FOR HEPATITIS C

AME Assisted Special Issuance (AASI) is a process that provides Examiners the ability to re-issue an airman medical certificate under the provisions of an Authorization for Special Issuance of a Medical Certificate (Authorization) to an applicant who has a medical condition that is disqualifying under Title 14 of the Code of Federal Regulations (14 CFR) part 67.

An FAA physician provides the initial certification decision and grants the Authorization in accordance with 14 CFR § 67.401. The Authorization letter is accompanied by attachments that specify the information that treating physician(s) must provide for the re-issuance determination. If this is a first time issuance of an Authorization for the above disease/condition, and the applicant has all of the requisite medical information necessary for a determination, the Examiner must defer and submit all of the documentation to the AMCD or RFS for the initial determination.

Examiners may re-issue an airman medical certificate under the provisions of an Authorization, if the applicant provides the following:

- An Authorization granted by the FAA;
- Any symptoms the applicant has developed;
- The name and dosage of medication(s) used for treatment and/or prevention with comment regarding side effects; and
- A current liver function profile performed within the last 90 days.

The Examiner must defer to the AMCD or Region if:

- The applicant has developed symptoms;
- There has been a change in treatment regimen or the applicant has been placed on alpha-interferon;
- Any side effects from required medication; or
- An adverse change in liver function studies.

AASI FOR HYPERTHYROIDISM

AME Assisted Special Issuance (AASI) is a process that provides Examiners the ability to re-issue an airman medical certificate under the provisions of an Authorization for Special Issuance of a Medical Certificate (Authorization) to an applicant who has a medical condition that is disqualifying under Title 14 of the Code of Federal Regulations (14 CFR) part 67.

An FAA physician provides the initial certification decision and grants the Authorization in accordance with 14 CFR § 67.401. The Authorization letter is accompanied by attachments that specify the information that treating physician(s) must provide for the re-issuance determination. If this is a first time issuance of an Authorization for the above disease/condition, and the applicant has all of the requisite medical information necessary for a determination, the Examiner must defer and submit all of the documentation to the AMCD or RFS for the initial determination.

Examiners may re-issue an airman medical certificate under the provisions of an Authorization, if the applicant provides the following:

- An Authorization granted by the FAA current statement of the condition since last FAA medical examination;
- The name and dosage of medication(s) used for treatment and/or prevention with comment regarding side effects; and
- Current thyroid function studies performed within last 90 days.

The Examiner must defer to the AMCD or Region if:

- The applicant has developed hypothyroidism; or
- The thyroid function studies are elevated, suggesting inadequate treatment; or
- The applicant developed an associated illness, such as dysrhythmia.

AASI FOR HYPOTHYROIDISM

AME Assisted Special Issuance (AASI) is a process that provides Examiners the ability to re-issue an airman medical certificate under the provisions of an Authorization for Special Issuance of a Medical Certificate (Authorization) to an applicant who has a medical condition that is disqualifying under Title 14 of the Code of Federal Regulations (14 CFR) part 67.

An FAA physician provides the initial certification decision and grants the Authorization in accordance with 14 CFR § 67.401. The Authorization letter is accompanied by attachments that specify the information that treating physician(s) must provide for the re-issuance determination. If this is a first time issuance of an Authorization for the above disease/condition, and the applicant has all of the requisite medical information necessary for a determination, the Examiner must defer and submit all of the documentation to the AMCD or RFS for the initial determination.

Examiners may re-issue an airman medical certificate under the provisions of an Authorization, if the applicant provides the following:

- An Authorization granted by the FAA;
- The name and dosage of medication(s) used for treatment and/or prevention with comment regarding side effects;
- A statement regarding any other associated problems, such as cardiac or visual; and
- A statement regarding the current thyroid stimulating hormone (TSH) level performed within the last 90 days.

The Examiner should defer to the AMCD or Region if:

- The applicant develops a related problem in another system, such as cardiac; or
- The TSH level is elevated.

AASI FOR LYMPHOMA AND HODGKIN'S DISEASE

AME Assisted Special Issuance (AASI) is a process that provides Examiners the ability to re-issue an airman medical certificate under the provisions of an Authorization for Special Issuance of a Medical Certificate (Authorization) to an applicant who has a medical condition that is disqualifying under Title 14 of the Code of Federal Regulations (14 CFR) part 67.

An FAA physician provides the initial certification decision and grants the Authorization in accordance with 14 CFR § 67.401. The Authorization letter is accompanied by attachments that specify the information that treating physician(s) must provide for the re-issuance determination. If this is a first time issuance of an Authorization for the above disease/condition, and the applicant has all of the requisite medical information necessary for a determination, the Examiner must defer and submit all of the documentation to the AMCD or RFS for the initial determination.

Examiners may re-issue an airman medical certificate under the provisions of an Authorization, if the applicant provides the following:

- An Authorization granted by the FAA; and
- An update of the status of the disease from the last FAA medical examination and any testing deemed necessary by the treating physician.

The Examiner must defer to the AMCD or Region if:

- There has been any recurrence or disease progression
- Any new treatment is initiated

AASI FOR MELANOMA

AME Assisted Special Issuance (AASI) is a process that provides Examiners the ability to re-issue an airman medical certificate under the provisions of an Authorization for Special Issuance of a Medical Certificate (Authorization) to an applicant who has a medical condition that is disqualifying under Title 14 of the Code of Federal Regulations (14 CFR) part 67.

An FAA physician provides the initial certification decision and grants the Authorization in accordance with 14 CFR § 67.401. The Authorization letter is accompanied by attachments that specify the information that treating physician(s) must provide for the re-issuance determination. If this is a first time issuance of an Authorization for the above disease/condition, and the applicant has all of the requisite medical information necessary for a determination, the Examiner must defer and submit all of the documentation to the AMCD or RFS for the initial determination.

Examiners may re-issue an airman medical certificate under the provisions of an Authorization, if the applicant provides the following:

- An Authorization granted by the FAA, and
- A current status report performed within the last 90 days that must include all the required followup items and studies as listed in the Authorization letter and that confirms absence of recurrent disease

The Examiner must defer to the AMCD or Region if:

- There has been any recurrence of the cancer, or
- Any new treatment is initiated

Note:

* A Special Issuance or AASI is required for any metastatic melanoma regardless of Breslow level

* A Special Issuance or AASI is required for any melanoma which exhibits Breslow Level > .75 mm with or without metastasis

* A melanoma that exhibits a Breslow Level < .75 mm which has no evidence of metastasis may be regular issued.

AASI FOR METABOLIC SYNDROME

(Glucose Intolerance, Impaired Glucose Tolerance, Impaired Fasting Glucose, Insulin Resistance, and Pre-Diabetes)

AME Assisted Special Issuance (AASI) is a process that provides Examiners the ability to re-issue an airman medical certificate under the provisions of an Authorization for Special Issuance of a Medical Certificate (Authorization) to an applicant who has a medical condition that is disqualifying under Title 14 of the Code of Federal Regulations (14 CFR) part 67.

An FAA physician provides the initial certification decision and grants the Authorization in accordance with 14 CFR § 67.401. The Authorization letter is accompanied by attachments that specify the information that treating physician(s) must provide for the re-issuance determination. If this is a first time issuance of an Authorization for the above disease/condition, and the applicant has provided all of the requisite medical information necessary for a determination, the Examiner must defer and submit all of the documentation to the AMCD or RFS for the initial determination.

Examiners may re-issue an airman medical certificate under the provisions of an Authorization, if the applicant provides the following:

- An Authorization granted by the FAA;
- A statement attesting that the airman is maintaining his or her diabetic diet;
- A statement regarding any diabetic symptomatology; and
- The results of a current HgA1c level performed within last 90 days.

The Examiner must defer to the AMCD or Region if:

- The applicant has been placed on insulin;
- The HgA1c level is greater than 9.0 mg%
- Any hypoglycemic event
- The applicant has developed evidence of any of the following:
  - Cardiovascular disease,
  - Neurologic disease, including any change in degree of peripheral neuropathy,
  - Ophthalmologic disease,
  - Renal disease (including a Creatinine over 2.0)
- The airman has been placed on any amlynomimetics, such as pramlintide (Symlin)
- There is a change in oral hypoglycemic medication
- The airman has been placed on beta-blockers AND his/her oral diabetes medications include any sulfonlyurea and/or any meglitinide. **Commonly used meglitinides include repaglinide (Prandin) and nateglinide (Starlix). Commonly used sulfonylureas include: acetohexamide (Dymelor); chloropropamide (Diabinese); tolazamide (Tolinase); tolbutamide (Orinase); glimepiride (Amaryl); glipizide (Glucotrol, Glucotrol XL); glyburide (DiaBeta, Micronase, Glynase); glyburide plus metformin (Glucovance); glipizide plus metformin (Metaglip).**
- Any new treatment is initiated

AASI FOR MIGRAINES

AME Assisted Special Issuance (AASI) is a process that provides Examiners the ability to re-issue an airman medical certificate under the provisions of an Authorization for Special Issuance of a Medical Certificate (Authorization) to an applicant who has a medical condition that is disqualifying under Title 14 of the Code of Federal Regulations (14 CFR) part 67.

An FAA physician provides the initial certification decision and grants the Authorization in accordance with 14 CFR § 67.401. The Authorization letter is accompanied by attachments that specify the information that treating physician(s) must provide for the re-issuance determination. If this is a first time issuance of an Authorization for the above disease/condition, and the applicant has all of the requisite medical information necessary for a determination, the Examiner must defer and submit all of the documentation to the AMCD or RFS for the initial determination.

Examiners may re-issue an airman medical certificate under the provisions of an Authorization, if the applicant provides the following:

- An Authorization granted by the FAA;
- A statement regarding the frequency of headaches and/or other associated symptoms since last followup report;
- A statement regarding if the characteristics of the headaches changed; and
- The name and dosage of medication(s) used for treatment and/or prevention with comment regarding side effects.

The Examiner must defer to the AMCD or Region if:

- The frequency of headaches and/or other symptoms increase since the last followup report; or
- The applicant is placed on medication(s), such as isometheptene mucate, narcotic analgesic, tramadol, tricyclic-antidepressant medication, etc.

AASI FOR MITRAL OR AORTIC INSUFFICIENCY

AME Assisted Special Issuance (AASI) is a process that provides Examiners the ability to re-issue an airman medical certificate under the provisions of an Authorization for Special Issuance of a Medical Certificate (Authorization) to an applicant who has a medical condition that is disqualifying under Title 14 of the Code of Federal Regulations (14 CFR) part 67.

An FAA physician provides the initial certification decision and grants the Authorization in accordance with 14 CFR § 67.401. The Authorization letter is accompanied by attachments that specify the information that treating physician(s) must provide for the re-issuance determination. If this is a first time issuance of an Authorization for the above disease/condition, and the applicant has all of the requisite medical information necessary for a determination, the Examiner must defer and submit all of the documentation to the AMCD or RFS for the initial determination.

Examiners may re-issue an airman medical certificate under the provisions of an Authorization, if the applicant provides the following:

- An Authorization granted by the FAA;
- A summary of the applicant's medical condition since the last FAA medical examination, including a statement regarding any further episodes of atrial fibrillation; and
- A current 2-D echocardiogram with Doppler performed within the last 90 days.

The Examiner must defer to the AMCD or Region if:

- The mean gradient across the valve reaches 40 mm HG;
- New symptoms occur;
- An arrhythmia develops; or
- The treating physician or Examiner reports the murmur is now moderate to severe (Grade III or IV).

AASI FOR PAROXYSMAL ATRIAL TACHYCARDIA

AME Assisted Special Issuance (AASI) is a process that provides Examiners the ability to re-issue an airman medical certificate under the provisions of an Authorization for Special Issuance of a Medical Certificate (Authorization) to an applicant who has a medical condition that is disqualifying under Title 14 of the Code of Federal Regulations (14 CFR) part 67.

An FAA physician provides the initial certification decision and grants the Authorization in accordance with 14 CFR § 67.401. The Authorization letter is accompanied by attachments that specify the information that treating physician(s) must provide for the re-issuance determination. If this is a first time issuance of an Authorization for the above disease/condition, and the applicant has all of the requisite medical information necessary for a determination, the Examiner must defer and submit all of the documentation to the AMCD or RFS for the initial determination.

Examiners may re-issue an airman medical certificate under the provisions of an Authorization, if the applicant provides the following:

- An Authorization granted by the FAA;
- A statement regarding any recurrences since the last FAA medical examination; and
- The name and dosage of medication(s) used for treatment and/or prevention with comment regarding side effects.

The Examiner must defer to the AMCD or Region if:

- There have been one or more recurrences; or
- The applicant has received some treatment that was not reported in the past, such as radiofrequency ablation

AASI FOR PROSTATE CANCER

AME Assisted Special Issuance (AASI) is a process that provides Examiners the ability to re-issue an airman medical certificate under the provisions of an Authorization for Special Issuance of a Medical Certificate (Authorization) to an applicant who has a medical condition that is disqualifying under Title 14 of the Code of Federal Regulations (14 CFR) part 67.

An FAA physician provides the initial certification decision and grants the Authorization in accordance with 14 CFR § 67.401. The Authorization letter is accompanied by attachments that specify the information that treating physician(s) must provide for the re-issuance determination. If this is a first time issuance of an Authorization for the above disease/condition, and the applicant has all of the requisite medical information necessary for a determination, the Examiner must defer and submit all of the documentation to the AMCD or RFS for the initial determination.

Examiners may re-issue an airman medical certificate under the provisions of an Authorization, if the applicant provides the following:

- An Authorization granted by the FAA;
- A current status of the medical condition to include any testing deemed necessary; and
- A current PSA level performed within the last 90 days.

The Examiner must defer to the AMCD or Region if:

- The PSA rises at a rate above 0.75 ng/ml per year;
- A new treatment is initiated; or
- Any metastasis has occurred.

AASI FOR RENAL CALCULI

AME Assisted Special Issuance (AASI) is a process that provides Examiners the ability to re-issue an airman medical certificate under the provisions of an Authorization for Special Issuance of a Medical Certificate (Authorization) to an applicant who has a medical condition that is disqualifying under Title 14 of the Code of Federal Regulations (14 CFR) part 67.

An FAA physician provides the initial certification decision and grants the Authorization in accordance with 14 CFR § 67.401. The Authorization letter is accompanied by attachments that specify the information that treating physician(s) must provide for the re-issuance determination. If this is a first time issuance of an Authorization for the above disease/condition, and the applicant has all of the requisite medical information necessary for a determination, the Examiner must defer and submit all of the documentation to the AMCD or RFS for the initial determination.

Examiners may re-issue an airman medical certificate under the provisions of an Authorization, if the applicant provides the following:

- An Authorization granted by the FAA;
- A statement from your treating physician regarding the location of the retained stone(s), estimation as to size of stone, and likelihood of becoming symptomatic; and
- A current report of appropriate imaging study (IVP, KUB, Ultrasound, or Spiral CT Scan) and provide a metabolic work-up, both performed within the last 90 days.

The Examiner must defer to the AMCD or Region if:

- If the treating physician comments that the current stone has a likelihood of becoming symptomatic;
- If the retained stone(s) has moved when compared to previous evaluations; or
- If the stone(s) has become larger when compared to previous evaluations.

AASI FOR RENAL CARCINOMA

AME Assisted Special Issuance (AASI) is a process that provides Examiners the ability to re-issue an airman medical certificate under the provisions of an Authorization for Special Issuance of a Medical Certificate (Authorization) to an applicant who has a medical condition that is disqualifying under Title 14 of the Code of Federal Regulations (14 CFR) part 67.

An FAA physician provides the initial certification decision and grants the Authorization in accordance with 14 CFR § 67.401. The Authorization letter is accompanied by attachments that specify the information that treating physician(s) must provide for the re-issuance determination. If this is a first time issuance of an Authorization for the above disease/condition, and the applicant has all of the requisite medical information necessary for a determination, the Examiner must defer and submit all of the documentation to the AMCD or RFS for the initial determination.

Examiners may re-issue an airman medical certificate under the provisions of an Authorization, if the applicant provides the following:

- An Authorization granted by the FAA; and
- A current status report performed within the last 90 days that must include all the required followup items and studies as listed in the Authorization letter and that confirms absence of recurrent disease.

The Examiner must defer to the AMCD or Region if:

- There has been any recurrence of the cancer; or
- Any new treatment is initiated.

AASI FOR SLEEP APNEA

AME Assisted Special Issuance (AASI) is a process that provides Examiners the ability to re-issue an airman medical certificate under the provisions of an Authorization for Special Issuance of a Medical Certificate (Authorization) to an applicant who has a medical condition that is disqualifying under Title 14 of the Code of Federal Regulations (14 CFR) part 67.

An FAA physician provides the initial certification decision and grants the Authorization in accordance with 14 CFR § 67.401. The Authorization letter is accompanied by attachments that specify the information that treating physician(s) must provide for the re-issuance determination. If this is a first time issuance of an Authorization for the above disease/condition, and the applicant has all of the requisite medical information necessary for a determination, the Examiner must defer and submit all of the documentation to the AMCD or RFS for the initial determination.

Examiners may re-issue an airman medical certificate under the provisions of an Authorization, if the applicant provides the following:

- An Authorization granted by the FAA; and
- A current report (performed within the last 90 days) from the treating physician that references the present treatment, whether this has eliminated any symptoms and with specific comments regarding daytime sleepiness. If there is any question about response to or compliance with treatment, then a Maintenance of Wakefulness Test (MWT) will be required.

The Examiner must defer to the AMCD or Region if:

- There is any question concerning the adequacy of therapy;
- The applicant appears to be non-compliant with therapy;
- The MWT demonstrates sleep deficiency; or
- The applicant has developed some associated illness, such as right-sided heart failure.

AASI FOR TESTICULAR CARCINOMA

AME Assisted Special Issuance (AASI) is a process that provides Examiners the ability to re-issue an airman medical certificate under the provisions of an Authorization for Special Issuance of a Medical Certificate (Authorization) to an applicant who has a medical condition that is disqualifying under Title 14 of the Code of Federal Regulations (14 CFR) part 67.

An FAA physician provides the initial certification decision and grants the Authorization in accordance with 14 CFR § 67.401. The Authorization letter is accompanied by attachments that specify the information that treating physician(s) must provide for the re-issuance determination. If this is a first time issuance of an Authorization for the above disease/condition, and the applicant has all of the requisite medical information necessary for a determination, the Examiner must defer and submit all of the documentation to the AMCD or RFS for the initial determination.

Examiners may re-issue an airman medical certificate under the provisions of an Authorization, if the applicant provides the following:

- An Authorization granted by the FAA; and
- A current status report performed within the last 90 days that must include all the required followup items and studies as listed in the Authorization letter and that confirms absence of recurrent disease.

The Examiner must defer to the AMCD or Region if:

- There has been any recurrence of the cancer; or
- Any new treatment is initiated.

AASI FOR WARFARIN (COUMADIN) THERAPY FOR DEEP VENOUS THROMBOSIS (DVT), PULMONARY EMBOLISM (PE), AND/ OR HYPERCOAGULOPATHIES

AME Assisted Special Issuance (AASI) is a process that provides Examiners the ability to re-issue an airman medical certificate under the provisions of an Authorization for Special Issuance of a Medical Certificate (Authorization) to an applicant who has a medical condition that is disqualifying under Title 14 of the Code of Federal Regulations (14 CFR) part 67.

An FAA physician provides the initial certification decision and grants the Authorization in accordance with 14 CFR § 67.401. The Authorization letter is accompanied by attachments that specify the information that treating physician(s) must provide for the re-issuance determination. If this is a first time issuance of an Authorization for the above disease/condition and the applicant has all of the required medical information necessary for a determination, the Examiner must defer and submit all of the documentation to the AMCD or RFS for the initial determination.

Examiners may re-issue an airman medical certificate under the provisions of an Authorization, if the applicant provides the following:

- An Authorization granted by the FAA;
- A summary of the applicant's medical condition since the last FAA medical examination, including a statement regarding any further episodes of DVT, PE or other complication of hypercoagulopathy (see below*);
- The name and dosage of medication(s) used for treatment and/or prevention with comment regarding side effects; and
- A minimum of monthly International Normalized Ratio (INR) results for the immediate prior 6 months (see below*).

* The Examiner must defer to the AMCD or Region if:

- More than 20 percent of INR values are <2.0 or >3.0; or
- The applicant develops emboli, thrombosis, bleeding that required medical intervention, or any other cardiac or neurologic condition previously not diagnosed or reported.

AME Assisted Special Issuance (AASI) for Third-Class Airman Medical Certificate

AME Assisted Special Issuance (AASI) is a process that provides Examiners the ability to re-issue an airman medical certificate under the provisions of an Authorization for Special Issuance of a Medical Certificate (Authorization) to an applicant who has a medical condition that is disqualifying under Title 14 of the Code of Federal Regulations (14 CFR) part 67.

The AASI's listed below are presently restricted to the issue of a **third-class** airman medical certificate.

An FAA physician provides the initial certification decision and grants the Authorization in accordance with 14 CFR § 67.401. The Authorization letter is accompanied by attachments that specify the information that treating physician(s) must provide for the re-issuance determination. If this is a first time issuance of an Authorization for the above disease/condition, and the applicant has all of the requisite medical information necessary for a determination, the Examiner must defer and submit all of the documentation to the AMCD or RFS for the initial determination.

For **Third-class:**

> Coronary Heart Disease (to include):
> Angina Pectoris
> Atherectomy
> Brachytherapy
> Coronary Bypass Grafting
> Myocardial Infarction
> Percutaneous Transluminal Angioplasty (PTCA)
> Rotoblation
> Stent Insertion
>
> Valve Replacement

AASI FOR CORONARY HEART DISEASE

AME Assisted Special Issuance (AASI) is a process that provides Examiners the ability to reissue an airman medical certificate to an applicant who has a medical condition that is disqualifying under Title 14 of the Code of Federal Regulations, (14 CFR) part 67. This AASI is presently restricted to the issue of a **third-class** airman medical certificate for an applicant with a history of Angina Pectoris; Atherectomy; Brachytherapy; Coronary Bypass Grafting; Myocardial Infarction; Percutaneous Transluminal Angioplasty (PTCA); Rotoblation; or Stent Insertion. First- and second-class applicants must be deferred to the FAA.

The FAA physicians provide the initial certification decision and grant the Authorization for Special Issuance of a Medical Certificate (Authorization) in accordance with 14 CFR § 67.401. The Authorization letter is accompanied by attachments that specify the information that treating physician(s) must provide for the issuance determination. If this is a first time issuance of an Authorization for the above disease/condition, and the airman has all of the requisite medical information necessary for a determination, you must defer and submit all of the documentation to the AMCD or your RFS for the initial determination.

Examiners may reissue an airman medical certificate if the applicant provides the following:

- An Authorization granted by the FAA;
- A current status report performed within the past 90 days in accordance with the CHD Protocol; and
- A current maximal GXT – See GXT Protocol

The Examiner must defer medical certification to AMCD or Region if:

- The applicant complains of chest pain at any time (exclude chest pain with a firm diagnosis of non-cardiac causes of chest pain);
- The applicant has another event (myocardial infarction, or restenosis requiring CABG, atherectomy, brachytherapy, PTCA, or stent);
- The applicant for whatever reason is placed on a long acting nitrate;
- The applicant's risk factors are inadequately controlled; or
- Has any reason for not renewing an AASI – See GXT Protocol; or
- The applicant develops bleeding that required medical intervention or other cardiac condition not previously diagnosed or reported.

AASI FOR SINGLE VALVE REPLACEMENT

AME Assisted Special Issuance (AASI) is a process that provides Examiners the ability to re-issue an airman medical certificate under the provisions of an Authorization for Special Issuance of a Medical Certificate (Authorization) to an applicant who has a medical condition that is disqualifying under Title 14 of the Code of Federal Regulations (14 CFR) part 67.

This AASI is presently restricted to the issue of a **third-class** airman medical certificate. First- and second-class applicants must be deferred to the FAA. An FAA physician provides the initial certification decision and grants the Authorization in accordance with 14 CFR § 67.401. The Authorization letter is accompanied by attachments that specify the information that treating physician(s) must provide for the re-issuance determination. If this is a first time issuance of an Authorization for the above disease/condition, and the applicant has all of the requisite medical information necessary for a determination, the Examiner must defer and submit all of the documentation to the AMCD or RFS for the initial determination.

Examiners may re-issue an airman medical certificate under the provisions of an Authorization, if the applicant provides the following:

- An Authorization granted by the FAA
- A current status report performed within the past 90 days in accordance with the CHD Protocol
- A current 2D echocardiogram performed within 90 days
- For Mechanical Heart Values - A minimum of monthly International Normalized Ratio (INR) results for the immediate prior six months

The Examiner must defer medical certification to AMCD or Region if:

- The airman requires another valve procedure
- Evidence of perivalvular leaking via echocardiogram
- The post procedure valve area is less than 1.0 cm^2
- New onset arrhythmia such as of atrial fibrillation/flutter, ventricular bigeminy, ventricular tachycardia, Mobitz Type II or greater AV block, complete heart block, RBBB, LBBB or LVH
- More than 20% of INR values are less than 2.5 or greater than 3.5. In select cases of a Bileaflet (St. Jude) valve in the aortic position, INR values between 2.0 and 3.0 may be accepted (check with FAA)
- The applicant reports any other disqualifying medical condition or undergoes therapy not previously reported
- The applicant develops emboli, thrombosis, bleeding that required medical intervention, or any other cardiac condition previously not diagnosed or reported

Aviation Medical Examiner
Assisted Special Issuance (AASI)
Certificate Issuance

I have reviewed the enclosed medical report(s) and have determined that the report(s) is in accordance with this applicant's Authorization for Special Issuance of a Medical Certificate and the AASI Protocol established for certificate issuance.

I have issued a _____ -class medical certificate to the airman named below with all other limitations listed on the original certificate. The certificate issued is timed limited by the restriction "NOT VALID FOR ANY CLASS AFTER _____ "

Date

Check all that apply:

☐ Interim certificate issued for disease(s)/condition(s) below – No examination performed.

ALL	AASI CONDITION	ALL	AASI CONDITION	ALL	AASI CONDITION
	Arthritis		Metabolic Syndrome, Glucose Intolerance, Impaired Glucose Tolerance, Impaired Fasting Glucose, Insulin Resistance, and Pre-Diabetes		Prostate Cancer
	Asthma		Glaucoma		Renal Calculi
	Atrial Fibrillation		Hepatitis C		Renal Cancer
	Bladder Cancer		Hyperthyroidism		Sleep Apnea
	Breast Cancer		Hypothyroidism		Testicular Cancer
	Chronic Lymphocytic Leukemia		Lymphoma and Hodgkins		Warfarin (Coumadin) Therapy for Deep Venous Thrombosis, Pulmonary Embolism, and/ or Hypercoagulopathies.
	Chronic Obstructive Pulmonary		Melanoma		
	Colitis (Ulcerative or Crohn's)		Migraine Headaches		
	Colon Cancer		Mitral and Aortic Insufficiency		
	Diabetes Mellitus – Type II Medication Controlled		Paroxysmal Atrial Tachycardia		
THIRD CLASS ONLY	AASI CONDITION			**THIRD CLASS ONLY**	
	Coronary Heart Disease				

☐ Certificate issued - New application and examination performed.

AIRMAN INFORMATION:

Name:

PI: DOB:

AVIATION MEDICAL EXAMINER (AME) INFORMATION:

AME Name (Print):

AME Signature:

AME Number: Date:

SUBSTANCES OF DEPENDENCE/ABUSE

LAST UPDATE: December 14, 2012

Substances of Dependence/Abuse

As an Examiner you are required to be aware of the regulations and Agency policy and have a responsibility to inform airmen of the potential adverse effects of medications and to counsel airmen regarding their use. There are numerous conditions that require the chronic use of medications that do not compromise aviation safety and, therefore, are permissible. Airmen who develop short-term, self-limited illnesses are best advised to avoid performing aviation duties while medications are used.

Aeromedical decision-making includes an analysis of the underlying disease or condition and treatment. The underlying disease has an equal and often greater influence upon the determination of aeromedical certification. It is unlikely that a source document could be developed and understood by airmen when considering the underlying medical condition(s), drug interactions, medication dosages, and the shear volume of medications that need to be considered. A list may encourage or facilitate an airmen's self-determination of the risks posed by various medical conditions especially when combination therapy is used. A list is subject to misuse if used as the sole factor to determine certification eligibility or compliance with 14 CFR part 61.53, Prohibition of Operations During Medical Deficiencies. Maintaining a published a list of "acceptable" medications is labor intensive and in the final analysis only partially answers the certification question and does not contribute to aviation safety.

Therefore, the list of medications referenced provides aeromedical guidance about specific medications or classes of pharmaceutical preparations and is applied by using sound aeromedical clinical judgment. This list is not meant to be totally inclusive or comprehensive. No independent interpretation of the FAA's position with respect to a medication included or excluded from the following should be assumed. See Aviation Industry Antidrug and Alcohol Misuse Prevention Programs

Substances of Dependence/Abuse

ALCOHOL DEPENDENCE/ABUSE

AMPHETAMINES

ANXIOLYTICS

COCAINE

HYPNOTICS

HALLUCINOGENS

MARIJUANA

NARCOTICS

PHENCYCLIDINE (PCP)

PSYCHOTROPIC

STIMULANTS

TRANQUILIZERS

The following is applicable to each Substances of Dependence/Abuse referenced above:

I. CODE OF FEDERAL REGULATIONS
First-Class Airman Medical Certificate: 67.107
Second-Class Airman Medical Certificate: 67.207
Third-Class Airman Medical Certificate: 67.307

II. MEDICAL HISTORY and CONVICTIONS OR ADMINISTRATIVE ACTIONS.

Medical History: **Item 18.n.,** Substance dependence; or failed a drug test ever; or substance abuse or use of illegal substance in the last 2 years.

"Substance" includes alcohol and other drugs (e.g., PCP, sedatives and hypnotics, anxiolytics, marijuana, cocaine, opioids, amphetamines, hallucinogens, and other psychoactive drugs or chemicals). For a "yes" answer to Item 18.n., the Examiner should obtain a detailed description of the history. A history of substance dependence or abuse is disqualifying. The Examiner must defer issuance of a certificate if there is doubt concerning an applicant's substance use.

Convictions or Administrative Actions: **Item 18.v.**, Conviction and/or Administrative Action History

The events to be reported are specifically identified in Item 18.v. of FAA Form 8500-8. If "yes" is checked, the applicant must describe the conviction(s) and/or administrative action(s) in the EXPLANATIONS box. The description must include:

- The alcohol or drug offense for which the applicant was convicted or the type of administrative action involved (e.g., attendance at an educational or rehabilitation program in lieu of conviction; license denial, suspension, cancellation, or revocation for refusal to be tested; educational safe driving program for multiple speeding convictions; etc.);

- The name of the state or other jurisdiction involved; and
- The date of the conviction and/or administrative action

If there have been no new convictions or administrative actions since the last application, the applicant may enter "PREVIOUSLY REPORTED, NO CHANGE." Convictions and/or administrative actions affecting driving privileges may raise questions about the applicant's fitness for certification and may be cause for disqualification.

A single driving while intoxicated (DWI) conviction or administrative action usually is not cause for denial if there are no other instances or indications of substance dependence or abuse. The Examiner should inquire regarding the applicant's alcohol use history, the circumstances surrounding the incident, and document those findings in **Item 60.**

NOTE: The Examiner should advise the applicant that the reporting of alcohol or drug offenses (i.e., motor vehicle violation) on the history part of the medical application does not relieve the airman of responsibility to report each motor vehicle action to the FAA within 60 days of the occurrence to the Civil Aviation Security Division, AAC-700; P.O. Box 25810; Oklahoma City, OK 73125-0810.

III. AEROMEDICAL DECISION CONSIDERATIONS: See **Item 47.**, Psychiatric, Aerospace Medical Disposition table.

IV. PROTOCOL: See Substances of Dependence/Abuse Protocol

V. Aviation Industry Antidrug and Alcohol Misuse Prevention Programs

SYNOPSIS OF MEDICAL STANDARDS

SUMMARY OF MEDICAL STANDARDS – Revised April 3, 2006

Medical Certificate Pilot Type	First-Class Airline Transport Pilot	Second-Class Commercial Pilot	Third-Class Private Pilot
DISTANT VISION	20/20 or better in each eye separately, with or without correction.		20/40 or better in each eye separately, with or without correction.
NEAR VISION	20/40 or better in each eye separately (Snellen equivalent), with or without correction, as measured at 16 inches.		
INTERMEDIATE VISION	20/40 or better in each eye separately (Snellen equivalent), with or without correction at age 50 and over, as measured at 32 inches.		No requirement.
COLOR VISION	Ability to perceive those colors necessary for safe performance of airman duties.		
HEARING	Demonstrate hearing of an average conversational voice in a quiet room, using both ears at 6 feet, with the back turned to the examiner or pass one of the audiometric tests below.		
AUDIOLOGY	Audiometric speech discrimination test: Score at least 70% reception in one ear. Pure tone audiometric test. Unaided, with thresholds no worse than:		

	500 Hz	1,000 Hz	2,000 Hz	3,000 Hz
Better Ear	35 Db	30 dB	30 dB	40 dB
Worst Ear	35 dB	50 dB	50 dB	60 dB

ENT	No ear disease or condition manifested by, or that may reasonably be expected to maintained by, vertigo or a disturbance of speech or equilibrium.		
PULSE	Not disqualifying per se. Used to determine cardiac system status and responsiveness.		
BLOOD PRESSURE	No specified values stated in the standards. The current guideline maximum value is 155/95.		
ELECTRO-CARDIOGRAM (ECG)	At age 35 and annually after age 40	Not routinely required.	
MENTAL	No diagnosis of psychosis, or bipolar disorder, or severe personality disorders.		
SUBSTANCE DEPENDENCE AND SUBSTANCE ABUSE	A diagnosis or medical history of "substance dependence" is disqualifying unless there is established clinical evidence, satisfactory to the Federal Air Surgeon, of recovery, including sustained total abstinence from the substance(s) for not less than the preceding 2 years. A history of "substance abuse" within the preceding 2 years is disqualifying. "Substance" includes alcohol and other drugs (i.e., PCP, sedatives and hynoptics, anxiolytics, marijuana, cocaine, opioids, amphetamines, hallucinogens, and other psychoactive drugs or chemicals).		
DISQUALIFYING CONDITIONS	Unless otherwise directed by the FAA, the Examiner must deny or defer if the applicant has a history of: (1) Diabetes mellitus requiring hypoglycemic medication; (2) Angina pectoris; (3) Coronary heart disease that has been treated or, if untreated, that has been symptomatic or clinically significant; (4) Myocardial infarction; (5) Cardiac valve replacement; (6) Permanent cardiac pacemaker; (7) Heart replacement; (8) Psychosis; (9) Bipolar disorder; (10) Personality disorder that is severe enough to have repeatedly manifested itself by overt acts; (11) Substance dependence; (12) Substance abuse; (13) Epilepsy; (14) Disturbance of consciousness and without satisfactory explanation of cause, and (15) Transient loss of control of nervous system function(s) without satisfactory explanation of cause.		

NOTE: For further information, contact your Regional Flight Surgeon.

GLOSSARY

GLOSSARY/ACRONYMS

AAM - Office of Aerospace Medicine

AASI - AME Assisted Special Issuance - Criteria under which an Examiner may reissue a medical certificate for a third-class applicant with a medical history of a disqualifying condition, who has already received a Special Issuance Authorization from the FAA, and criteria to defer issuance to AMCD or RFS for these situations.

AMCD - Aerospace Medical Certification Division - located at the Civil Aerospace Medical Institute in Oklahoma City, Oklahoma

AMCS - Airman Medical Certification System - allows the AME to electronically submit FAA Form 8500-8, Application for Airman Medical Certificate or Airman Medical and Student Pilot Certificate, to AMCD.

AME - Aviation Medical Examiner - a physician designated by the FAA and given the authority to perform airman physical examinations for issuance of second- and third-class medical and student pilot certificates. (NOTE: Senior Examiners perform first-class airman examinations).

ATCS - Air Traffic Control Specialist

AV - Atrioventricular

BUN - Blood Urea Nitrogen Test

CAD - Coronary Artery Disease

CAMI - Civil Aerospace Medical Institute

CAT - Computerized Axial Tomography Scan

CBC - Complete Blood Count

CEA - Carcinoembryonic Antigen

CFR - Code of Federal Regulations

CHD - Coronary Heart Disease

CT - Computed Tomography Scan

CVE - Cardiovascular Evaluation

DOT - Department of Transportation

DUI/DWI - Driving Under The Influence/Driving While Intoxicated

ECG - Electrocardiogram

ECHO - Echocardiographic images

ENT - Ear, Nose, and Throat

FAA - Federal Aviation Administration

FAR - Federal Aviation Regulations

FSDO - Flight Standards District Office

GXT - Graded Exercise Test

HgbA1C - Hemoglobin A1C

INR- International Normalized Ratio

IVP - Intravenous Pyelography Test

KUB - Kidneys, Ureters and Bladder

MFO - Medical Field Office

MFT - Medical Flight Test

MRI - Magnetic Resonance Imaging

MVP - Mitral Valve Prolapse

NTSB - National Transportation Safety Board

PAC's - Premature Arterial Contractions

PET - Radioactive High-Tech Scan

PFT - Pulmonary Function Test

PSA - Prostate Specific Antigen

PT - Prothrombin Time

PTT - Partial Thromboplastin Time

PVC's - Premature Ventricular Contractions

RF - Radio Frequency Ablation

RFS - Regional Flight Surgeon

SODA - Statement of Demonstrated Ability

TFT -Thyroid Function Test

US -Ultrasound

ARCHIVES AND MODIFICATIONS

LAST UPDATE: December 14, 2012

				of the Requirement for **Individuals Granted the Special Issuance of a Medical Certificate To Carry Their Letter of Authorization While Exercising Pilot Privileges**," references to the requirement to carry an LOA were removed from the General Information and Special Issuances sections of the Guide.
2012	07/03/12	1.	Medical Policy	In Item 41. G-U System, remove information on "Contraceptives and Hormone Replacement Therapy." Move this information to a new page of the same title within the Pharmaceuticals section.
2012	06/30/12	1.	Medical Policy	In Item 41. G-U System, create new section for pregnancy.
2012	06/07/12	1.	Medical Policy	In Item 41. G-U System, revise guidance on Gender Identity Disorder to specify requirements for current status report, psychiatric and/or psychological evaluations, and surgery follow-up reports.
2012	05/25/12	1.	Medical Policy	In Item 52. Color Vision, add chart for criteria and acceptable tests for Air Traffic Controllers (FAA employee 2152 series and Contract Tower ATCS).
2012	01/31/12	1.	Medical Policy	In Decision Considerations. Aerospace Medical Dispositions, Item 45. Lymphatics, revise title from 'Hodgkin's Disease – Lymphoma" to "Lymphoma and Hodgkin's Disease."
2012	01/26/12	1.	Medical Policy	In Examination Techniques. Item 48. Hypothyroidism, add note that AMES may call FAA for verbal clearance if airman presents current lab reports.
		2.	Medical Policy	In Pharmaceuticals, Allergy – Desensitization Injections, Change the title and

				references to Allergy – Immunotherapy. Add note stating that sublingual immunotherapy (SLIT) is not acceptable.
		3.	Medical Policy	In Examination Techniques, Item 36. Heart, remove requirement for reporting serum potassium values if the airman is taking diuretics.
		4.	Medical Policy	In Protocol for Evaluation of Hypertension, remove requirement for reporting serum potassium if the airman is taking diuretics.
		5.	Medical Policy	In Item 36. Heart – Dispositions Table, Coronary Artery Disease, revise table to clarify evaluation data required for third class.
2012	01/03/12	1.	Administrative	Revise cover page to reflect the current calendar year.
		2.	Medical Policy	In General Information, Medical Certificates – AME Completion, revise language to clarify signature requirements.
2011	12/13/11	1.	Medical Policy	In Examination Techniques, Item 52. Color Vision, revise to include Color Vision Testing Flowchart.
2011	12/01/11	1.	Medical Policy	In Pharmaceuticals (Therapeutic Medications) section, change title of Antihistaminic and Desensitization Injections to include the word "Allergy." Also, change title of Diabetes Mellitus – Type II Medication Controlled to include "(Non Insulin)." This title was also changed in the AASI.
		2.	Medical Policy	In Pharmaceuticals (Therapeutic Medications) Acne Medications, revise page format to clarify policy.
2011	11/16/11	1.	Medical Policy	In General Information, Disposition of Applications and Medical Examinations, Clarify to indicate that Student Pilot

				Applications and Examinations must be transmitted to AMCD within 7 days.
2011	11/01/11	1.	Medical Policy	In Pharmaceuticals – Insulin, revise to clarify guidance on medication combinations.
2011	10/24/11	1.	Administrative	In Aerospace Medical Dispositions, Item 49. Hearing, clarify guidance on hearing aids.
2011	09/15/11	1.	Medical Policy	In Examination Techniques, Item 31 – 34. Eye - Orthokeratology, revise to clarify policy.
		2.	Medical Policy	In Aerospace Medical Dispositions, Item 31. Eyes – General, revise to include information on Keratoconus.
		3.	Medical Policy	In General Information, Equipment Requirements, revise to include equipment to measure height and weight.
2011	09/12/11	1.	Medical Policy	In Aerospace Medical Dispositions, Item 47., Psychiatric Conditions – Use of Antidepressants, include SSRI Specification Sheet for guidance.
		2.	Medical Policy	In Pharmaceuticals, Antidepressants, revise to clarify medical history, protocol, and pharmaceutical considerations.
		3.	Administrative	In Table of Contents, renumber entries listed on pages iii and iv.
2011	08/12/11	1.	Medical Policy	In Special Issuances, Third-Class AME Assisted – Valve Replacement, revise to include additional criteria for deferral ("the applicant develops emboli, thrombosis, etc.").
		2.	Medical Policy	In Special Issuances, AME Assisted – All Classes – Atrial Fibrillation, revise to include additional criteria for deferral ("bleeding that required medical intervention").
		3.	Medical Policy	In Special Issuances, AME Assisted – All Classes –

				Warfarin (Coumadin) Therapy for Deep Venous Thrombosis (DVT), Pulmonary Embolism (PE), and/ or Hypercouagulopathies, revise to include additional criteria for deferral ("bleeding that required medical intervention").
		4.	Medical Policy	In Special Issuances, Third-Class AME Assisted – Coronary Heart Disease, revise to include additional criteria for deferral ("bleeding that required medical intervention").
2011	08/09/11	1.	Medical Policy	In Disease Protocols, Coronary Heart Disease, correct in item A.1.b., "replacement" to "repair."
		2.	Administrative	In Pharmaceuticals – Antihypertensive, revise to clarify unacceptable medications.
		3.	Administrative	In Examination Techniques, Item 36., Heart, revise to clarify unacceptable medications.
		4.	Administrative	In Aerospace Medical Dispositions, Item 55., revise to clarify blood pressure limits.
		5.	Administrative	In Aerospace Medical Dispositions, Item 47., Psychiatric Conditions, revise table to include information on depression requiring the use of antidepressant medications.
		6.	Administrative	In Disease Protocols, Hypertension, revise to clarify unacceptable medications.
2011	05/25/11	1.	Administrative	In Examination Techniques, Item 47., Psychiatric, revise SSRI Follow Up Chart to clarify procedure.
2011	05/08/11	1.	Administrative	In Pharmaceuticals, reorganize and clarify the page content for Acne Medications, Antacids, Anticoagulants, Antihistaminic, Antihypertensive,

				Desensitization Injections, Diabetes – Type II Medication Controlled, Glaucoma Medications, and Insulin.
2011	03/11/11	1.	Medical Policy	In Aerospace Medical Dispositions, Item 47., Psychiatric Conditions, clarify policy verbiage on Bipolar Disorder and Psychosis.
2011	03/02/11	1.	Medical Policy	In Aerospace Medical Dispositions, Item 47., Psychiatric Conditions, add section titled "Use of Antidepressant Medication," to state revised policy on use of SSRIs.
2011	02/23/11	1.	Medical Policy	In Aerospace Medical Dispositions, Item 52., Color Vision, clarify pass criterion for OPTEC 900 Vision Tester.
2011	02/03/11	1.	Medical Policy	In Medical History, Item 18. v., History of Arrest(s), Conviction(s), and/ or Administrative Action(s), reorder, revise, and clarify deferral and issuance criteria.
2011	01/31/11	1.	Errata	Revise to correct transposed words in title: Decision Considerations, Disease Protocols – "Graded Exercise Stress Test – Bundle Branch Block Requirements."
2011	01/07/11	1.	Administrative	Revise cover page to reflect current calendar year.
2010	11/23/10	1.	Medical Policy	In Exam Techniques, Item 26. Nose and Item 35. Lungs and Chest, revise and clarify criteria for hay fever medications.
		2.	Medical Policy	In Pharmaceuticals (Therapeutic Medications) - Desensitization Injections, revise and clarify criteria for hay fever medications.
2010	10/29/10	1.	Medical Policy	In Aerospace Medical Dispositions, Item 52. Color Vision, remove Titmus II Vision Tester (Model Nos. TII and TIIS) as an acceptable substitute for color vision

				testing.
2010	09/20/10	1.	Medical Policy	In AASI Protocol for Arthritis, change title to "Arthritis and/ or Psoriasis." Clarify authorization and deferral criteria.
2010	09/03/10	1.	Medical Policy	In Exam Techniques, Item 21-22 Height and Weight, add Body Mass Index Chart and Formula Table.
2010	06/15/10	1.	Medical Policy	In Aerospace Medical Dispositions, Item 48, General Systemic, clarify disposition for Hyperthroydism and Hypothyrodism. First Special Issuance requires FAA decision. Guidance for Followup Special Issuance is found in AASI Protocol.
		2.	Administrative	In AASI Protocol for Hyperthyroidism and Protocol for Hypothyroidism, clarify criteria for deferring and issuing.
2010	05/20/10	1.	Administrative	In Aerospace Medical Dispositions, Item 47, Psychiatric Conditions Table of Medical Dispositions, clarify "see below" information in Evaluation Data column.
2010	03/17/10	1.	Medical Policy	In Disease Protocols, Binocular Multifocal and Accommodating Devices, clarify criteria for adaptation period before certification.
		2.	Medical Policy	In Applicant History, Item 17b, revise and clarify criteria regarding use of types of contact lenses.
		3.	Medical Policy	In Exam Techniques, Items 31-34 Eye – Contact Lenses, revise and clarify criteria.
2010	01/20/10	1.	Administrative	Revise cover page to reflect current calendar year.
		2.	Medical Policy	In Applicant History, Item 18 Medical History, v. History of Arrest(s), Conviction(s), and/or Administrative Action(s), revise and clarify deferral and issuance criteria.

2009	12/08/09	1.	Medical Policy	In Examination Techniques, Item 52. Color Vision, remove APT-5 as an acceptable color vision tester.
2009	10/22/09	1.	Medical Policy	In Examination Techniques, Item 52. Color Vision, add note to Agency-Designated AMEs: "Not all tests approved for pilots are acceptable for FAA ATCSs. Contact RFS for current list."
2009	10/16/09	1.	Medical Policy	In Special Issuance, Diabetes Mellitus – Type II, Medication Controlled, revise to reflect further criteria required for AME re-issuance: current status report from physician treating diabetes to include any history of hypoglycemic events and any cardiovascular, renal, neurologic or opththalmologic complications; and HgA1c level performed within the last 30 days.
2009	09/30/2009	1.	Medical Policy	In Disease Protocols, Diabetes Mellitus – Type I or Type II, Insulin Treated, add note to indicate that insulin pumps are acceptable.
		2.	Medical Policy	In Disease Protocols, revise main listing to reflect addition of "Diabetes Mellitus and Metabolic Syndrome – Diet Controlled" and "Metabolic Syndrome (Glucose Intolerance, Impaired Glucose tolerance, Impaired Fasting Glucose, Insulin Resistance, and Pre-Diabetes) - Medication Controlled."
		3.	Medical Policy	In Aerospace Medical Dispositions, Item 48. General Systemic – Diabetes, Metabolic Syndrome, and/or Insulin Resistance, revise table to reflect addition of "Diabetes Mellitus and Metabolic Syndrome – Diet Controlled" and "Metabolic

				Syndrome (Glucose Intolerance, Impaired Glucose tolerance, Impaired Fasting Glucose, Insulin Resistance, and Pre-Diabetes) - Medication Controlled."
		4.	Medical Policy	In Disease Protocols, add new protocol outlining Metabolic Syndrome, Medication Controlled.
		5.	Medical Policy	In Disease Protocols, Diabetes Mellitus – Diet Controlled, revise to reflect Diabetes Mellitus and Metabolic Syndrome (Glucose Intolerance, Impaired Glucose tolerance, Impaired Fasting Glucose, Insulin Resistance, and Pre-Diabetes) - Diet Controlled
2009	09/21/2009	1.	Errata	In Disease Protocols, Substances of Dependence/Abuse (Drugs and Alcohol), change "personnel statement" to "personal statement."
		2.	Medical Policy	In Special Issuance, Colon Cancer; Chronic Lymphocytic Leukemia; Diabetes Mellitus – Type II, Medication Controlled; and Lymphoma and Hodgkin's Disease, add if "Any new treatment is initiated" – to criteria for deferment to AMCD or Region.
		3.	Medical Policy	In Aerospace Medical Dispositions, Item 48. General Systemic, Diabetes – change title to "Diabetes, Metabolic Syndrome, and/or Insulin Resistance." Also add new table entry to reflect criteria for "Metabolic Syndrome or Insulin Resistance."
		4.	Medical Policy	In AME Assisted Special Issuance, All Classes – added entry and criteria for Metabolic Syndrome (Glucose Intolerance, Impaired Glucose Tolerance, Impaired Fasting

				Glucose, Insulin Resistance, and Pre-Diabetes). Also added entry on AASI Certificate Issuance sheet.
		5.	Administrative	In General Information, Who May Be Certified, b. Language Requirements – added information to clarify guidance on certification and reporting process.
2009	07/30/2009	1.	Medical Policy	In Pharmaceuticals, Acne Medications, add language to further clarify instructions for deferral and restrictions.
2009	07/09/2009	1.	Medical Policy	In Pharmaceuticals, Diabetes Mellitus – Type II, Medication Controlled, revise to remove amlynomimetics from allowable combinations.
		2.	Medical Policy	In AASI, Diabetes Mellitus – Type II, Medication Controlled, revise criteria for deferring to AMCD or region.
2009	05/13/2009	1.	Medical Policy	In General Information, Equipment Requirements and Examination Equipment and Techniques, Item 52. Color Vision, add OPTEC 2500 as acceptable vision testing substitute.
2009	04/30/2009	1.	Errata	In Examination Techniques, Item 31-34. Eye, correct typographical error in form number. Revised to reflect "8500-7."
2009	04/24/2009	1.	Medical Policy	In AASI, Diabetes Mellitus – Type II, Medication Controlled; and Pharmaceuticals, Diabetes Mellitus - Type II, Medication Controlled - revise to clarify criteria for deferring to AMCD or region also to clarify allowable medication combinations.
2009	02/04/2009	1.	Administrative	Revise cover page to reflect current calendar year.
2008	12/11/2008	1.	Medical Policy	In Examination Techniques, Item 52. Color Vision, revise language to specify that AME-administered aviation Signal

					Light Gun test is prohibited.
2008	10/30/2008	1.		Errata	In Examination Techniques and Aerospace Medical Dispositions, Item 52. Color vision, revise to list correct testing plates for Richmond HRR, 4th Edition.
2008	10/10/2008	1.		Administrative	In General Information, create new section 12. "Medical Certificates – AME Completion."
		2.		Administrative	In Table Of Contents, General Information, adjust and renumber listings to reflect inclusion of Medical Certificates – AME Completion.
		3.		Medical Policy	In Examination Techniques, Item 52., Color Vision, add new vision tester.
		4.		Medical Policy	In Aerospace Medical Disposition, Item 52. Color Vision, revise section A., All Classes, to include standard for new vision tester.
2008	09/17/2008	1.		Medical Policy	Change Applicant History, 18. v. Conviction and/or Administrative Action History to "History of Arrest(s), Conviction(s), and/or Administrative Action(s). Revise language within 18. v. to include reference to arrests.
		2.		Medical Policy	Revise Applicant History to create a new section, 18.y. Medical Disability Benefits.
		3.		Medical Policy	Revise Entire Guide to replace any usage of term "Urinalysis" with "Urine Test(s)."
2008	09/05/2008	1.		Administrative	Change cover page to remove "Version V" title. Change title to reflect current calendar year.
		2.		Medical Policy	In General Information, Equipment Requirements, and in Examination Techniques Items 50, 51, and 54, revise acceptable vision testing equipment requirements.
		3.		Medical Policy	In Aerospace Medical

				Dispositions, Item 52., Color Vision, revise to provide guidance on Specialized Operational Medical Tests: the Operational Color Vision Test and the Medical Flight Test. Also, update list of acceptable and unacceptable color vision testing equipment.
V.	07/31/2008	1.	Medical Policy	In General Information, Equipment Requirements, and in Examination Techniques (Items 50-52 and 54), revise acceptable vision testing equipment.
V.	07/16/2008	1.	Medical Policy	In General Information, Validity of Medical Certificates, revise third-class duration standards for airmen under age 40.
		2.	Medical Policy	In General Information, Requests for Assistance, revise to remove references to international and military examiners.
		3.	Administrative	In General Information, Classes of Medical Certificates, revise to clarify "flying activities" to "privileges."
		4.	Medical Policy	In Special Issuances, revise to include language requiring airman to carry Authorization when exercising pilot privileges.
		5	Medical Policy	In Applicant History, Guidance for Positive Identification of Airmen, revise to include link to 14 CFR §67.4. Applicants must show proof of age and identity.
V.	04/1/2008	1.	Administrative	In General Information, Who May Be Certified, add guidance on ICAO standard for English Proficiency, Operational Level 4.
		2.	Medical Policy	In General information, Equipment Requirements, revise list of acceptable equipment, particularly acceptable substitute

				equipment for vision testing.
		3.	Medical Policy	In Exam Techniques, Item 50, Distant Vision, revise equipment list of acceptable substitutes.
		4.	Medical Policy	In Exam Techniques, Item 51. Near and Intermediate Vision, revise equipment table of acceptable substitutes.
		5.	Medical Policy	In Exam Techniques, Item 54. Heterophoria, revise equipment table of acceptable substitutes.
V.	02/01/2008	1.	Medical Policy	In Exam Techniques, Item. 52. Color Vision, revise Section E., which clarifies unacceptable tests.
V.	01/11/2008	1.	Medical Policy	In AME Assisted Special Issuance (AASI), add section on Warfarin (Coumadin) Therapy for Deep Venous Thrombosis, Pulmonary Embolism, and/ or Hypercoagulopathies.
		2.	Medical Policy	Revise AASI coversheet to include box for Warfarin (Coumadin) Therapy for Deep Venous Thrombosis, Pulmonary Embolism, and/ or Hypercoagulopathies.
V.	11/26/2007	1.	Administrative	In General Information, Validity of Medical Certificates, delete note for "Flight outside the airspace of the United States of America."
		2.	Administrative	In Disease Protocols, Conductive Keratoplasty (CK), revise description of CK procedure.
		3.	Errata	In Aerospace Medical Dispositions, Item 31. Eye, correct typographical error.
		4.	Medical Policy	In Pharmaceuticals, add "Malaria Medications."
V.	11/26/2007	5.	Medical Policy	In Exam Techniques, Item 51. Near and Intermediate vision, add Keystone Orthoscope and Keystone Telebinocular.

		6.	Administrative	In Airman Certification Forms, add note regarding International Standards on Personnel Licensing.
		7.	Administrative	In General Information, Equipment Requirements, add note regarding the possession and maintenance of equipment.
		8.	Administrative	In General Information, Privacy of Medical Information, add note on the protection of privacy information.
		9.	Administrative	In General Information, Disposition of Applications, add note to include electronic submission by international AME's.

V.	11/26/2007	10.	Medical Policy	In Exam Techniques and Criteria, 31-34 Eye, Refractive Procedures, revise to include Wavefront-guided LASIK.
V.	09/01/2007	1.	Administrative	Revise title of Disease Protocols, "Antihistamines" to "Allergies, Severe."
		2.	Administrative	In Pharmaceuticals, add "Acne Medications" and "Glaucoma Medications."
		3.	Medical Policy	Add policy regarding use of isotretinoin (Accutane) in Pharmaceuticals; Aerospace Medical Dispositions, Item 40. Skin; and Examination Techniques and Criteria for Qualification, Item. 40 Skin
		4.	Errata	Revise Protocol for Maximal Graded Exercise Stress Test Requirements to change "8 minutes" to "9 minutes."
		5.	Errata	In Aerospace Medical Dispositions, Item. 36. Heart – Atrial Fibrillation - change "CHD Protocol with ECHO and 24-hour Holter" to read "See CVE Protocol with EST, Echo, and 24-hour Holter."
		6.	Medical Policy	Revise Aerospace Medical Dispositions, Item 36. Heart - Syncope.
		7.	Medical Policy	Revise Examination Techniques and Criteria for Qualification, Item. 36 Heart – Auscultation.

Guide Version	Official Date	Revision Number	Description Of Change	Reason For Modification
V.	09/01/2007	8.	Administrative	In Pharmaceuticals, Antihypertensive, V. Pharmaceutical Considerations – remove "D. AME Assisted – All Classes, Atrial Fibrillation."
		9.	Administrative	In Pharmaceuticals, Antihistaminic, V. Pharmaceutical Considerations – add "C. Aerospace Medical Dispositions, Item 35. Lungs and Chest."
		10.	Medical Policy	Revise Disease Protocols, Coronary Heart Disease to clarify requirements for consideration for any class of airman medical certification.
		11.	Errata	Revise Disease Protocols, Coronary Heart Disease to remove "Limited to Flight Engineer Duties."
V.	04/25/2007	1.	Administrative	Move Leukemia, Acute and Chronic from Aerospace Medical Dispositions Item 48. General Systemic to Item 48. General Systemic, Blood and Blood-Forming Tissue Disease.

Guide Version	Official Date	Revision Number	Description Of Change	Reason For Modification
V.	04/25/2007	2.	Administrative	Revise Aerospace Medical Dispositions Item 48. General Systemic to include disposition table titled "Neoplasms."
		3.	Administrative	Move Breast Cancer from Aerospace Medical Dispositions Item 38. Abdomen and Viscera - Malignancies to Item 48. General Systemic, Neoplasms. Also, move Colitis (Ulcerative, Regional Enteritis or Crohn's disease) and Peptic Ulcer from Aerospace Medical Dispositions Item 38. Abdomen and Viscera – Malignancies to Item 38. Abdomen and Viscera and Anus Conditions.
		4.	Administrative	Update individual Pharmaceutical pages to include "Pharmaceutical Considerations."
V.	11/20/2006	1.	Medical Policy	Insert into Disease Protocols a new section on Cardiac Transplant for Class III certificates only.
		2.	Errata	Corrected AASI on Mitral or Aortic Insufficiency to read "mean gradient."

Guide Version	Official Date	Revision Number	Description Of Change	Reason For Modification
V.	08/23/2006	1.	Errata	INR values for mechanical valves should have read between 2.5 and 3.5, except for certain types of bileaflet valves in the aortic position.
		2.	Administrative	Clarified the Hypertension Protocol regarding initiation and change of medication and the suspension of pilot duties.
		3.	Errata	Maximal graded exercise stress test requirement for under age 60 corrected to 9 minutes.
		4.	Medical Policy	Remove prohibition on bifocal contact lenses or lenses that correct for near and/or intermediate vision in Items 31-34, Eyes; Section 5, Contact Lenses.
		5.	Medical Policy	Update Neurological Conditions Disposition Table and Footnote #21 with guidance on Rolandic Seizure.
		6.	Administrative	Clarified language in General Information, Item 9. Who May Be Certified; a. Age Requirements.

Archives and Modifications

Guide Version	Official Date	Revision Number	Description Of Change	Reason For Modification
V.	04/03/2006	1.	Administrative	Redesign the appearance and navigable format of the *Guide for Aviation Medical Examiners*
		2.	Administrative	Install a Search Engine located in the Navigation Bar
		3.	Administrative	Revise Heading Titles for Chapters 2, 3, and 4
		4.	Administrative	Insert a Special Issuances section located in the Navigation Bar and into the General Information section
		5.	Administrative	Insert a Policy Updates section to post new and revised Administrative and Medical Policies
		6.	Medical Policy	Insert into the AME Assisted Special Issuance (AASI) section a Testicular Carcinoma AASI
		7.	Medical Policy	Revise Atrial Fibrillation AASI
		8.	Medical Policy	Revise Asthma AASI
		9.	Medical Policy	Revise Hyperthyroidism and Hypothyroidism AASIs
		10.	Medical Policy	Insert a new AASI subsection containing Coronary Heart Disease and Single Valve Replacement applicable for Third-Class only

Archives and Modifications

Guide Version	Official Date	Revision Number	Description Of Change	Reason For Modification
V.	04/03/2006	11.	Medical Policy	Insert into the Disease Protocols section a new Coronary Heart Disease and Graded Exercise Stress Test Protocol, and revise the Valve Replacement Protocol
		12.	Administrative	Insert Items 49 – 58 into the Examination Techniques section
		13.	Medical Policy	Revise Item 35. Lungs and Chest, Asthma, Aerospace Medical Disposition Table
		14.	Medical Policy	Revise Item 36. Heart, Atrial Fibrillation, Aerospace Medical Disposition Table
		15.	Medical Policy	Revise Item 36. Heart, Coronary Heart Disease, Aerospace Medical Disposition Table
		16.	Medical Policy	Revise Item 36. Heart, Valvular Disease, Aerospace Medical Disposition Table
		17.	Medical Policy	Revise Item 48. General Systemic, Hyperthyroidism and Hypothyroidism, Aerospace Medical Disposition Table
		18.	Medical Policy	Revise all Oral Medications - Diabetes Mellitus, Type II references
		19.	Medical Policy	Revise FAA Form 8500-7, Report of Eye Evaluation

Guide Version	Official Date	Revision Number	Description Of Change	Reason For Modification
IV.	07/31/2005	1.	Administrative	Redesign the appearance and navigable format of the *Guide for Aviation Medical Examiners*
		2.	Administrative	Revise Section 9., Refractive Surgery heading in Items 31-34. Eyes, to Refractive Procedures
		3.	Medical Policy	Insert Conductive Keratoplasty into Section 9, Items 31-34, Eyes, and into Item 31's Aerospace Medical Disposition Table
		4.	Administrative	Replace optometrist or ophthmologist reference(s) to "eye specialist"
		5.	Medical Policy	Insert Pulmonary Embolism into Item 35, Lungs and Chest, Aerospace Medical Disposition Table
		6.	Medical Policy	Insert Deep Vein Thrombosis and Pulmonary Embolism into Item 37, Vascular System, Aerospace Medical Disposition Table
		7.	Medical Policy	Insert Deep Vein Thrombosis and Pulmonary Embolism into the Thromboembolic Protocol.

Guide Version	Official Date	Revision Number	Description Of Change	Reason For Modification
IV.	01/16/2006	8.	Medical Policy	Insert into the Disease Protocol section a Conductive Keratoplasty Protocol
		9.	Medical Policy	Delete a paragraph located in Item 31-34. EYE, Section 4. Monocular vision
		10.	Medical Policy	Insert into the Disease Protocol section a Binocular Multifocal and Accommodating Devices Protocol
		11.	Medical Policy	Insert into the AME Assisted Special Issuance (AASI) section the new Bladder, Breast, Melanoma, and Renal Carcinoma AASI's
III.	11/01/2004	1.	Medical Policy	Revise AASI Process to include First- and Second-class Airman Medical Certification
		2.	Administrative	Insert into General Information, a new Section 10 that provides Sport Pilot Provisions
		3.	Administrative	Update revised Title 14, Code of Federal Regulations, §61.53
		4.	Administrative	Insert a link to download a revised AME Letter of Denial
		5.	Administrative	Insert a link to download a printable AASI Certificate Coversheet

Guide Version	Official Date	Revision Number	Description Of Change	Reason For Modification
II.	02/13/2004	1.	Administrative	Install Search Engine located in the Navigation Bar
		2.	Administrative	Insert a WHAT'S NEW link located in the Navigation Bar
		3.	Administrative	The "Instructions" site of the 2003 Guide is deleted and incorporated into the "Introduction" and "Available Downloads" located in the Navigation Bar
		4.	Administrative	Insert an "Available Downloads" site located in the Navigation Bar
		5.	Administrative	Insert a Table of Contents and an Index into the pdf version of the 2004 Guide
		6.	Administrative	Insert a one-page synopsis of the Medical Standards located in the Navigation Bar
		7.	Medical Policy	Insert Section 6. Orthokeratology into Items 31-34. Eye
		8.	Administrative	Relocate Item 46. Footnote # 21 from Head Trauma to Footnote #19, Headaches
		9.	Administrative	Insert Attention Deficit Disorder into Item 47's, Aerospace Medical Disposition Table
		10.	Medical Policy	Revise Item 60; Comments on History and Findings
		11.	Medical Policy	Revise Item 63; Disqualifying Defects
		12.	Medical Policy	Delete from AASI's a History of Monocularity
		13.	Administrative	Insert an Archives located in the Navigation Bar
	09/16/2004	14.	Administrative	Insert CAD Ultrasound into Item 37's, Aerospace Medical Disposition Table
I.	09/24/2003	Introduction of the 2003 Guide for Aviation Medical Examiners Website		

www.ingramcontent.com/pod-product-compliance
Lightning Source LLC
Chambersburg PA
CBHW081109170526
45165CB00008B/2382